Map Key

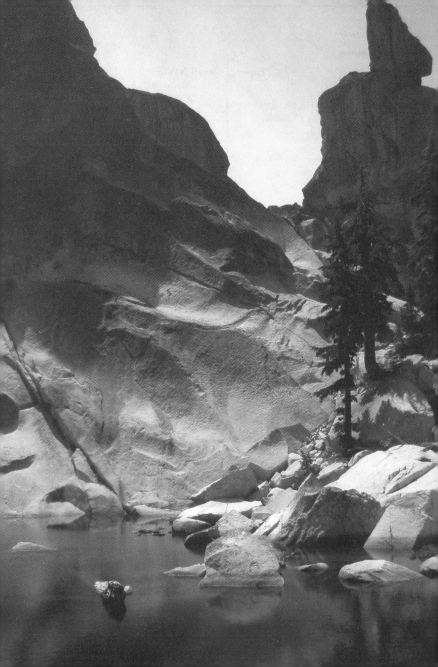

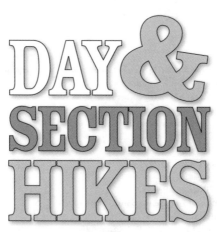

DAY & SECTION HIKES

Pacific Crest Trail
NORTHERN
CALIFORNIA

WENDY LAUTNER

 WILDERNESS PRESS ... *on the trail since 1967*

Day & Section Hikes Pacific Crest Trail: Northern California

1st EDITION 2010
   3rd printing 2015

Front cover photograph © 2010 by Wendy Lautner (main) and Greg Speicher (inset)
Interior photographs by Wendy Lautner
Maps by Scott McGrew and Wendy Lautner
Cover design by Scott McGrew
Book design by Ian Szymkowiak/Palace Press International

ISBN 978-0-89997-507-8

Manufactured in the United States of America

Published by: **Wilderness Press**
                2204 First Avenue South, Suite 102
                Birmingham, AL 35233
                (800) 443-7227; FAX (205) 326-1012
                info@wildernesspress.com
                www.wildernesspress.com

Visit our website for a complete listing of our books and for ordering information.
Distributed by Publishers Group West

Cover photos:	*Main:* Round Top (10,381 feet) towers above Winnemucca and Round Top lakes south of Carson Pass (Hike 10). *Inset:* Author Wendy Lautner climbs about 1000 feet in elevation on the way to Little Elk Lake (Hike 29).
Frontispiece:	Art gallery or the great outdoors? The backdrop at Statue Lake (Hike 27) will make you wonder.

SAFETY NOTICE: Although Wilderness Press and the author have made every attempt to ensure that the information in this book is accurate at press time, they are not responsible for any loss, damage, injury, or inconvenience that may occur to anyone while using this book. You are responsible for your own safety and health while in the wilderness. The fact that a trail is described in this book does not mean that it will be safe for you. Be aware that trail conditions can change from day to day. Always check local conditions, know your own limitations, and consult a map.

Table of Contents

PART 3: NORTH
INTERSTATE 80 TO PARADISE LAKE   III

*To everyone—veteran hikers and newbies alike—
who wishes to explore this beautiful place we call
the Pacific Crest Trail in Northern California*

*To Greg Speicher, without whose love and support
writing this book would not have been possible*

Acknowledgments

I MUST BEGIN BY ACKNOWLEDGING my first editor at Menasha Ridge Press, Russell Helms, who offered me the amazing opportunity to spend the better part of the past year hiking around Northern California and call it work. Russell, I can't thank you enough for offering me such an incredible "job." I must also thank my second editor at Menasha Ridge, Molly Merkle, whose editing expertise, thoughtful questions, and perspective greatly improved the content of my hike descriptions. Her friendliness and positive attitude helped ease the stress associated with finishing a book. I am deeply grateful as well to author Jeffrey Schaffer, whose books on the Pacific Crest Trail helped me immensely with my research.

While hiking and writing are second nature to me, mapping is not (despite that geography degree from Humboldt State University). I owe the accuracy and detail of these maps to Menasha Ridge cartography guru Scott McGrew and also to my father, Ben Lautner, who spent one very long day with me at the computer working out the bugs of my GPS unit and mapping software. My dad's curiosity about and interest in all that I do have been a driving force in helping me complete this book, and to him I am forever grateful. My mom, Carol Lautner, has also been an enormous fountain of inspiration; without her creative license on life and the dreams she instilled in me as a child (while we took long walks on the beaches of Lake Michigan), I may never have realized this dream.

In addition, I'd like to thank the following hiking and trail-running gurus who shared their expertise: Rachael Woods, who works at Alpine Meadows Ski Resort and spends her summers running around on the trails near Lake Tahoe; "Squarrel," who gave me advice on packing light; Kate Reid, who recommended that I add Clark Fork to the Disaster Creek hike (page 45); Alejandro Salazar, who recommended the Warren Lake hike (page 112); Joe Bosquin, who suggested that I include the trail into the Grand Canyon of the Tuolumne (page 31); and all the helpful rangers I met along the way.

Finally, I'd like to thank my trail partners: my sister, Sandra Parkhurst; Kelly Boire; Mali; Carson; and, most of all, my right-hand man and the love of my life, Greg Speicher. Not only did he join me on almost every step of my journey in researching this book, but his curiosity, undying support, and zest for life made this project one of the most amazing experiences of my life. Thank you so much, Greg.

Preface

THE PACIFIC CREST TRAIL WAS DESIGNATED as one of the first National Scenic Trails way back in 1968. As it traverses the "high road" from Mexico to Canada, incredible views are not only commonplace but also uniquely diverse, because the trail connects six of North America's seven eco-zones. The PCT's familiar, well-worn path is a special place for hikers from all walks of life on walks of all lengths and for all reasons.

In my travels on the PCT and surrounding connector trails throughout Northern California, I've often envied the strength and dedication of the 300 or so folks who attempt to hike its 2,650 miles each year. And as I've wandered into the PCT's more remote regions, I've pondered the footprints this path has seen and the handful of thru-hikers who have actually placed one foot in front of the other day after day, from Mexico to Canada. (If you're interested in thru-hiking the PCT in Northern California, check out *Pacific Crest Trail: Northern California, From Tuolumne Meadows to the Oregon Border* by Jeffrey P. Schaffer.)

I freely admit that I'm not in the same league as these hikers. How many of us would be willing to hike all day and sleep on the ground all night for four or five months straight? Are there ways to experience the trail without that kind of commitment?

The answer is an unqualified yes. Instead of guiding you through the arduous task of hiking the entire PCT, the goal of this book is to help you plan trips that incorporate hiking on the PCT in Northern California, whether you have just an afternoon to spare or you want to escape for the entire weekend. And because I'm sucker for scenery and a lake lover at heart, my hike choices most often include the opportunity for a wilderness swim or a summit hike to take in outstanding views. This cargo-pocket guide offers advice to help you make the most of your time away from civilization, however long (or short) that stretch may be.

Please enjoy yourself on the trail and make memories with your family and friends that will last a lifetime. But also remember to tread lightly and respect the incredible, often fragile natural environment therein. When you travel off-trail, do so only in small groups. Don't feed the wildlife. Obey all laws on the trail. Be careful when you're using matches. And by all means, pack out all the trash you've packed in, and help out everyone by picking up trash on the trail that is not yours. Above all, remember that you're a guest in one of the greatest kingdoms in the world—a natural kingdom far superior to the artificial world.

Recommended Hikes

RECOMMENDED HIKES

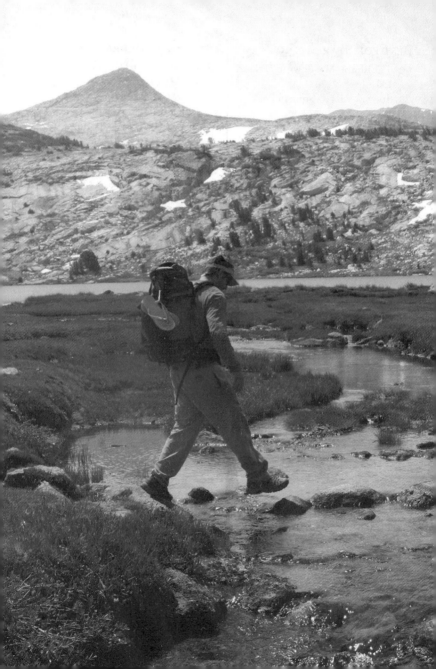

Introduction

How to Use This Guidebook

THE OVERVIEW MAP AND OVERVIEW MAP KEY

USE THE OVERVIEW MAP on the inside front cover to pinpoint the exact location of each hike's primary trailhead. Hike numbers appear on the overview map, on the map key facing the overview map, in the table of contents, at the beginning of each hike profile, and at the top of each trail map.

The book is organized by region as indicated in the table of contents, and the hikes within each region are noted as day hikes, overnight hikes, or a combination of the two. They are also labeled on the Table of Contents as out-and-back, loop, or point-to-point routes. A legend on the inside back cover explains the symbols found on the trail maps.

TRAIL MAPS

Each hike contains a detailed map that shows the trailhead, the route, significant features, facilities, and landmarks such as creeks, overlooks, and peaks. I gathered map data by carrying a Garmin eTrex Legend and Garmin eTrex Venture HC while hiking. This data was downloaded into a digital mapping program, TOPO USA, and then processed by an expert cartographer to produce the highly accurate maps in this book. Each trailhead's GPS coordinates are included with each profile (see page 2). In each hike's summary information, I also recommend a commercially available, color map that you may find useful, particularly for backpacking or cross-country trekking.

Crossing the outflow of an unnamed lake in Yosemite's high country on the way from Ireland Lake (Hike 2) to Vogelsang High Sierra Camp

ELEVATION PROFILES

Corresponding directly to the trail map, each hike contains an elevation profile that enables you to easily visualize how the trail rises and falls. Key points along the way are labeled. Note the number of feet between each tick mark on the vertical axis (the height scale). To keep flat hikes from looking steep and steep hikes from appearing flat, height scales are included to provide an accurate assessment of climbing difficulty.

GPS TRAILHEAD COORDINATES

To collect accurate map data, I carried a handheld GPS unit (Garmin eTrex series) as I scouted. The data collected was then downloaded and plotted onto a digital U.S. Geological Survey (USGS) topo map. In addition to rendering highly specific trail outlines, this book also includes the GPS coordinates for each trailhead in two formats: latitude–longitude and Universal Transverse Mercator (UTM). Latitude coordinates tell you where you are by locating points west of the zero-degree meridian line that passes through Greenwich; longitude coordinates do so by locating points north or south of the zero-degree line that belts the Earth, aka the equator.

Topographic maps show latitude and longitude data as well as UTM grid lines. Known as UTM coordinates, the numbers index a specific point using a grid method. The survey datum used to arrive at the coordinates in this book is WGS84 (versus NAD27 or WGS83). For readers who own a GPS unit, whether handheld or onboard a vehicle, the latitude–longitude or UTM coordinates provided on the first page of each hike may be entered into the GPS unit. Just make sure your GPS unit is set to navigate using WGS84 datum. Now you can navigate directly to the trailhead.

Most trailheads, which begin in parking areas, can be reached by car, but some hikes still require a short walk to reach the trailhead from a parking area. In those cases, a handheld unit is necessary to continue the GPS navigation process. That said, however, readers can easily access all trailheads in this book by using the directions given, the overview map, and the trail map, which shows at least one major road leading into the area. But for those who enjoy using the latest GPS technology to navigate, the necessary data has been provided. A brief explanation of the UTM coordinates from Warner Valley Road to Terminal Geyser (page 126) follows:

(page 126)

UTM Zone (WGS84) 10T
Easting 0635907
Northing 4478154

The zone number (10) refers to one of the 60 vertical zones of the UTM projection. Each zone is 6 degrees wide. The zone letter (T) refers to one of the 20 horizontal UTM zones that span from 80 degrees south to 84 degrees north. The easting number (0635907) indicates in meters how far east or west a point is from the central meridian of the zone. Increasing easting coordinates on a topo map or on your GPS screen indicate that you are moving east; decreasing easting coordinates indicate that you are moving west. The northing number (4478154) shows in meters how far you are from the equator. Above and below the equator, increasing northing coordinates indicate that you are traveling north; decreasing northing coordinates indicate that you are traveling south.

To learn more about how to enhance your outdoor experiences with GPS technology, refer to *Outdoor Navigation with GPS* by Stephen Hinch.

THE HIKE PROFILE

In addition to maps, each hike contains a concise but informative narrative of the hike from beginning to end. This descriptive text is enhanced with at-a-glance ratings and information, GPS-based trailhead coordinates, and accurate driving directions that lead you from a major road to the parking area most convenient to the trailhead.

At the beginning of each hike is a box that gives hikers quick access to pertinent information: quality of scenery, condition of the trail, the hike's appropriateness for children, the difficulty of the hike, the degree of solitude expected, hike distance, approximate hiking time, and outstanding highlights of the trip. The first five categories are rated using a five-star system. Below is an example:

26 Middle Deadfall Lake and Mount Eddy

SCENERY: ✿ ✿ ✿ ✿
TRAIL CONDITION: ✿ ✿ ✿ ✿ ✿
CHILDREN: ✿ ✿ ✿ ✿ ✿
DIFFICULTY: ✿
SOLITUDE: ✿ ✿
DISTANCE: *13.4 miles round-trip to the top*

of Mount Eddy and around Middle Deadfall Lake;
6 miles round-trip to Middle Deadfall Lake
HIKING TIME: *2–5 hours*
OUTSTANDING FEATURES: *Middle Deadfall*
Lake, wildflowers, views of Mount Shasta from
Mount Eddy

The four stars indicate that the scenery is very picturesque. The trail condition is excellent (one star would mean the trail is likely to be muddy, rocky, overgrown, or otherwise compromised). The hike is doable for able-bodied children (a one-star rating would denote that only the most gung-ho and physically fit children should go). The one star for difficulty lets you know that the hike is easy (five stars would be strenuous). The two stars for solitude mean you can expect to encounter some people on the trail (one star would mean you might well be elbowing your way past other hikers).

Distances given are absolute, but hiking times are estimated for an average hiking speed of 2 to 3 miles per hour, with time built in for pauses at overlooks and brief rests. Overnight-hiking times account for the effort of carrying a backpack.

Following each box is a brief italicized description of the hike. A more detailed account follows in which trail junctions, stream crossings, and trailside features are noted, along with their distance from the trailhead. Flip through the book, read the descriptions, and choose the hikes that appeal to you. The recommended hikes chart (see pages xii–xiii) also helps you choose a hike to fit your mood and group.

 # Weather

TEMPERATURE VARIATIONS in California are extreme. Folks in the Central Valley may very well be sweltering as the mercury easily passes the 100-degree mark in July and August. But on those very same days, the High Sierra can be downright frigid due to thunderstorms and high winds. The hikes described in this book range in elevation from around 2,000 feet at the Sacramento River outside Castle Crags State Park to 11,500 feet at the top of Sonora Peak. Pay careful attention to the elevations in which you'll be traveling, and plan accordingly. Thunderstorms in the High Sierra (anything above 6,000 feet) are especially common from July to October but can happen in any other month as well. Always pack a waterproof (or very water-resistant) shell, a warm layer (like fleece, *not* cotton), and a warm hat.

The summer hiking season, depending on snowfall, generally extends from early April to late October. But there's also a best time for every hike. For hikes set at the 5,000-foot elevation mark and under, wildflowers will be most abundant April through June. Hikes at this elevation are also good late-season hikes (October and November), depending on the current year's storm cycle.

For hikes above 5,000 feet, you'll have to watch the snowpack carefully to best time your hike. Generally, the trail is clear of substantial snowpack between the 5,000- and 8,000-foot elevation marks as summer rolls into late June; by July, the meadows and mountainsides between these elevations are covered in beautiful wildflowers. For hiking above the 8,000-foot mark, I recommend August because it is generally the warmest month and, if you're lucky, you'll catch the wildflowers and miss the mosquitoes. But never expect to be lucky. September is another perfect month to enjoy hiking above the 5,000-foot mark, but take note that the wildflowers will most likely be burned out below 8,000 feet (if not 10,000 feet). If you plan to exceed 10,000 feet in elevation, always expect to be cold no matter what month you're hiking. As a rule of thumb, the temperature decreases about three degrees with every 1,000 feet of elevation gained. And as you gain in elevation, the likelihood of wind increases also.

ALTITUDE SICKNESS

Nothing ruins an outing more often than the body's resistance to altitude adjustment. The illness is usually characterized by vomiting, loss of breath, extreme headache, lightheadedness, sleeplessness, and an overall sick feeling. When traveling to a higher altitude, give your body a day or two to adjust to where there is less oxygen, hotter sun, and less air pressure. Drink plenty of water, and lay off the alcohol. Wear sunglasses and sunscreen. It's that easy. (As always, if serious symptoms persist, locate the nearest emergency room or call 911.)

LIGHTNING

Get an early start on all hikes that go above tree line. Violent storms are common in June, July, and August. Try to reach high-altitude summits by 1 p.m. and turn back when the weather turns bad. If you are caught in a lightning storm above tree line, stay off ridgetops, spread out if you are in a group, and squat or sit on a foam pad with your feet together. Keep away from rock outcroppings and isolated trees. If someone has been struck, be prepared to use CPR to help restore the victim's breathing and heartbeat.

HYPOTHERMIA

Hypothermia occurs when your core body temperature becomes dangerously low. This condition can occur at any time of the year, and cold temperatures, wind, and rain and snow set the stage for complications. Look for signs of shivering, loss of coordination, and loss of judgment.

Preparation is your best defense against getting cold to the core. Remember the mantra "wet is not warm" to prevent hypothermia. Keep your inside layer as dry as possible.

Swift Water

Mountain streams can be dangerous during high snow runoff in May and June. Even a narrow stream may be deep and fast, as well as cold. Stay back from the banks of streams and rivers, especially if you cannot see the bottom. Provide proper supervision for children who tend to be attracted to water. Rocks at the streamside and in the stream are often slippery, and water beneath them may be deep. Powerful currents in streams can pull people underwater and pin them below the surface. In case of a flash flood, climb to safety.

Water

How much is enough? Well, one simple physiological fact should convince you to err on the side of excess when deciding how much water to pack: A hiker working hard in 90-degree heat needs approximately ten quarts of fluid per day. That's 2.5 gallons—12 large water bottles or 16 small ones. In other words, pack along one or two bottles even for short hikes.

Some hikers and backpackers hit the trail prepared to purify water found along the route. This method, while less dangerous than drinking it untreated, comes with risks. Purifiers with ceramic filters are the safest. Many hikers pack along the slightly distasteful tetraglycine-ñhydroperiodide tablets to debug water (sold under the names Potable Aqua, Coughlan's, and others). I have used the SteriPEN with excellent results. Lightweight, compact, and battery-operated, the device uses ultraviolet light to render harmful microbes sterile.

Probably the most common waterborne bug that hikers face is *giardia,* which may not hit until one to four weeks after ingestion. It will have you living in the bathroom, passing noxious rotten-egg gas, vomiting, and shivering with chills. Other parasites to worry about include *E. coli* and *cryptosporidium,* both of which are harder to kill than *giardia.*

For most people, the pleasures of hiking make carrying water a relatively minor price to pay to remain healthy. If you're tempted to drink found water, do so only if you understand the risks involved. Better yet, hydrate prior to your hike, carry (and drink) six ounces of water for every mile you plan to hike, and hydrate after the hike.

 # The Ten Essentials

ONE OF THE FIRST RULES OF HIKING is to be prepared for anything. The simplest way to be prepared is to carry the ten essentials. In addition to carrying the items listed below, you need to know how to use them, especially navigation items. Always consider worst-case scenarios like getting lost, hiking back in the dark, breaking gear (for example, a broken hip strap on your pack or a water filter getting clogged), twisting an ankle, or experiencing a brutal thunderstorm. The items listed below don't cost a lot of money, don't take up much room, and don't weigh much, but they just might save your life.

WATER: Durable bottles and water treatment such as iodine or a filter

MAP: Preferably a topo and a trail map with a route description

COMPASS: A high-quality model

FIRST-AID KIT: A good-quality kit whose contents you're familiar with and that contains instructions

KNIFE: Preferably a multitool device with pliers

LIGHT: Flashlight or headlamp with extra bulbs and batteries

FIRE: Windproof matches or lighter and fire starter

EXTRA FOOD: Always bring more than you need.

EXTRA CLOTHES: Rain protection, warm layers, gloves, and a warm hat

SUN PROTECTION: Sunglasses, lip balm, sunblock, and a sun hat

First-Aid Kit

A TYPICAL FIRST-AID KIT may contain more items than you might think necessary. These are just the basics. Prepackaged kits in waterproof bags (Atwater Carey and Adventure Medical make a variety of kits) are available. Even though there are quite a few items listed here, they pack down into a small space:

Ace bandages or Spenco joint wraps

Adhesive bandages

Antibiotic ointment (*Neosporin or the generic equivalent*)

Benadryl or the generic equivalent, diphenhydramine (*in case of allergic reactions*)

Butterfly-closure bandages

Epinephrine in a prefilled syringe (*for severe allergic reactions to bee stings, usually by prescription only*)

Gauze (*one roll*)

Gauze compress pads (*a half dozen 4 x 4-inch pads*)

Hydrogen peroxide or iodine

Ibuprofen or acetaminophen

Insect repellent

Matches or pocket lighter

Moleskin or Spenco Second Skin

Sunscreen

Whistle (*It's more effective at signaling rescuers than your voice is.*)

The following items are optional but worth their weight (make your own lists for different seasons and keep them in your hiking pack):

Aluminum foil

Bandana

Carabiners

Cellular phone (*emergencies only*)

Dark chocolate (*at least 60% cocoa*)

Digital camera

Disinfectant wipes (*baby wipes*)

Extra batteries

Flashlight

Foam pad (*for lightning strikes*)

Garbage bag

Gloves (*for warmth*)

GPS receiver

Hand warmers (*air activated*)

High-energy food and drinks

Lip balm

Long pants

Plastic bags with zip closure

Rain coat and rain pants

Shorts

Socks

Snakebite kit

Sunglasses

Toilet paper

Watch

General Safety

- **NO ONE IS TOO YOUNG FOR A HIKE.** Be mindful though. Flat, short, and shaded trails are best if you're carrying an infant. Toddlers who have not quite mastered walking can still tag along, riding on an adult's back in a child carrier. Use common sense to judge a child's capacity to hike a particular trail, and always expect that the child will tire quickly and need to be carried.

  Hiking is a great way to introduce a child to hands-on lessons beyond the classroom in the natural environment. Check out the top five hikes for children on page xiii.

- **NEVER RELY ON A CELL PHONE,** but bring one just in case. While signals and access are inconsistent, they are also becoming more common. A backcountry equestrian on the PCT turned me on to a very cool technology for keeping his wife informed of his whereabouts. Called SPOT GPS technology, it allows account holders' friends and family to constantly track carriers' whereabouts. The device features a help button that immediately sends coordinate locations to search and rescue professionals. Improvements are being made daily to allow users to upload pictures, videos, and so on that are tied to exact locations.

- **ALWAYS CARRY FOOD AND WATER,** whether you plan to go overnight or not. Food will give you energy, help keep you warm, and sustain you in an emergency until help arrives. You never know if you'll have a stream nearby when you become thirsty. Bring potable water, or treat water before drinking it from a stream. Boil or filter all found water before drinking it.

- **STAY ON DESIGNATED TRAILS.** Most hikers get lost when they leave the path. Even on the most clearly marked trails, there is usually a point where you have to stop and consider which direction to head in. If you become disoriented, don't panic. As soon as you think you may be off-track, stop, assess your current direction, and then retrace your steps to the point where you went awry. Using a map, a compass, and this book, and keeping in mind what you have passed thus far, reorient yourself and trust your judgment on how best to continue. If you become absolutely unsure of how to do so, return to your vehicle the same way you came in. If you become completely lost and have no idea how to return to the trailhead, stay where you are and wait for help—most often the best option for adults and always the best option for children.

· **BE ESPECIALLY CAREFUL WHEN CROSSING STREAMS.** Whether you are fording the stream or crossing on a log, make every step count. If you have any doubt about maintaining your balance on a foot log, go ahead and ford the stream instead. When crossing, use a trekking pole or stout stick for balance, and face upstream as you cross. If a stream seems too deep to ford, turn back. Whatever is on the other side is not worth risking your life for.

· **BE CAREFUL AT OVERLOOKS.** They may provide spectacular views, but they're potentially dangerous. Stay back from the edge of out-crops and be absolutely sure of your footing; a misstep can mean a nasty and possibly fatal fall.

· **STANDING DEAD TREES** and storm-damaged living trees pose a real hazard to hikers and tent campers. These trees may have loose or broken limbs that could fall at any time. When choosing a spot to rest or a backcountry campsite, look up.

· **TAKE ALONG YOUR BRAIN.** A cool, calculating mind is the single most important piece of equipment you can bring with you on the trail. Think before you act. Watch your step. Plan ahead. Avoid accidents before they happen.

Animal, Insect, and Plant Hazards

THE PACIFIC CREST TRAIL through Northern California is home to many species of wildlife. Insects such as mosquitoes, ticks, and flies are seasonally common on the trail. The most commonly seen mammals include deer, marmots, and squirrels, but it is not incon-ceivable to see a California black bear, especially in the Tuolumne Meadows area. You probably won't see mountain lions, but they are out there. Rattlesnakes are a hazard on sections of the PCT, gener-ally those areas under 6,000 feet. In the plant world, poison oak has a well-deserved nasty reputation and should be avoided at all costs.

And possibly the most dangerous things on the trail are microscopic waterborne organisms.

MOSQUITOES, TICKS, AND FLIES

Mosquitoes, ticks, and flies are the most common pitfalls of the PCT hiking experience, mosquitoes being the most plentiful of the three. Fortunately, the populations of these pests thins considerably after most of the standing water in an area has dried up.

Only female mosquitoes draw blood, proving my theory that females tend to work harder than males. The best protection is complete coverage if you're expecting to travel in mosquito-infested terrain—and on the PCT in the summer, you should expect this.

Bug-net trekking hats are incredibly useful at keeping mosquitoes out of your ears, eyes, nose, and mouth. Plus, nets that are attached to wide-brimmed hats keep the net away from your face and provide a less annoying screen through which you can enjoy the scenery.

When hiking in mosquito territory always carry light, loose, long layers. Zip-off pants are popular with many hikers. Leggings in the case of an emergency cover-up will not do the trick as many mosquitoes and/or flies can bite through leggings. Opt for light, loose-fitting, long layers to stave off itchy bites.

Keep in mind that mosquitoes on the PCT aren't so much dangerous as they are annoying. Some people choose to carry bug repellent containing DEET as a first-course step of treatment. Not only is DEET harmful to the environment, it's also harmful to apply directly to the skin and can ruin clothing. I recommend carrying bug dope only as a last resort. The Centers for Disease Control and Prevention considers the plant-based repellent lemon eucalyptus oil to be as effective in the same concentrations; plus it smells better and is safe to use on your skin and clothing.

Ticks tend to be most common in the densely forested areas below 4,000 feet north of the Lake Tahoe area on this section of the PCT. Check your clothing and skin after every hike for any hitchhiking ticks you may have acquired along the way. To remove a tick, grasp it as close to the skin's surface as possible with tweezers, and pull upward with steady, even pressure. Do not puncture a tick, as this might release harmful bacteria.

BLACK BEARS IN CALIFORNIA

An estimated 25,000 to 35,000 black bears call California home. They normally avoid humans, but you should always leave them an escape route if you encounter them. Black bears can sprint up to 35 mph and are strong swimmers and great tree climbers.

While these bears populate most of the area highlighted in this guidebook, the most common place to see bears on this section of the PCT is in the Tuolumne Meadows area in Yosemite National Park. Never leave scented products of any kind—food, beverages, or personal-care products such as lotion and sunscreen—in your vehicle unattended in the park area. The National Park Service provides unlocked communal lockers where hikers can store such items. Additionally, it is illegal to stay overnight in the backcountry in the Tuolumne Meadows area without a regulation bear canister, which you can buy or rent at the ranger station on Tioga Road.

MOUNTAIN LIONS

Mountain lion attacks on people are rare. Based on observations by people who have come in contact with mountain lions, some patterns are beginning to emerge. Here are more suggestions from the National Park Service:

- · STAY CALM.
- · TALK FIRMLY TO THE LION.
- · MOVE SLOWLY.
- · BACK UP OR STOP—NEVER RUN.
- · RAISE YOUR ARMS. If you are wearing a sweater or coat; open it and hold it wide.

- **PICK UP CHILDREN** to make them appear larger.

- **IF THE LION BECOMES AGGRESSIVE,** throw rocks and large objects at it. This is the time to convince the lion that you are not prey and that you are a danger to it.

- **NEVER CROUCH DOWN OR TURN YOUR BACK** to retrieve any belongings you may have dropped.

- **IF YOU ARE ATTACKED,** fight back and try to remain standing.

Rattlesnakes

The rattler is California's only venomous snake. The only known treatment for a bite is intravenous antivenom, which is only available at a hospital. If you are hiking alone and get bitten, calmly walk to where you can get help. If someone in your group has been bitten, send another person to get help quickly while the victim rests.

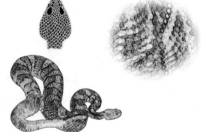

Rattlesnakes can be seen anywhere on or near the PCT and are most often spotted sunning themselves on warm rocks. Because they are nocturnal hunters, you will often see them at dusk. Always look before you reach, as most rattlers bite on the hand. Keep in mind that rattlers want to avoid confrontation and generally will alert you if you wander too close for their comfort.

Poison Oak

It has been said that poison oak is the one plight that keeps California from being perfect. Thankfully, you won't find much of it above 6,000 feet. Below 6,000 feet—that's another story. Most people have a strong allergic reaction to touching the plant and develop an

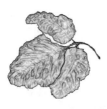

POISON OAK

extremely painful, itchy, bright-pink rash that most often consists of clusters of raised bumps. Some folks are more allergic than others, but there's no sense testing your possible immunity.

Recognize the tree/shrub by its clumps of three oak leaves. As the saying goes, "Leaves of three, let it be." In the spring and summer, the leaves often have an oily sheen; by late summer and/or early and late fall, they tend to turn bright red. If you think you've touched poison oak, wash the affected area with cold water immediately, and carry Tecnu (available at many outdoor stores) to treat clothes that may have brushed against it.

Tips for Enjoying the PCT in Northern California

FORTUNATELY, the scenery will likely cure any bad mood that might develop out on the trail. But here's some advice on things you can do to keep your smile.

· **PLAN FOR MORE TIME THAN YOU NEED.** The estimated times listed are for those who plan to travel at around 2 to 3 miles per hour. If you're planning to take lots of pictures, picnic breaks, and the like, build in much more time than the listed estimate. Also plan for more time than you think you'll need to drive to the trailhead. Many of these hikes have remote trailhead locations that require driving on unimproved roads.

· **SOLIDIFY THE NUTS AND BOLTS.** Are there fires in the area? Might some roads be closed due to snow? Will you need a permit to camp? A bear canister to pack in food? Call the local ranger district (see Appendix A, page 175) before you leave home.

· **PICK YOUR CAMPING/HIKING BUDDIES WISELY.** After you know who's going, make sure that everyone is on the same page regarding expectations of difficulty, sleeping arrangements, and food requirements. Also talk with your potential trail companions about their expectations of side activities—fishing, swimming, photography, and such—so that you can choose a hike that will suit everyone's needs.

- DON'T DUPLICATE EQUIPMENT such as cooking pots and lanterns among campers in your party. Carry what you need to have a good time, but don't turn the trip into a major moving experience.

- DRESS APPROPRIATELY FOR THE SEASON. Educate yourself on the highs and lows of the specific area you plan to visit. It may be warm at night in the summer in your backyard, but up in the mountains it can be quite chilly.

- PITCH YOUR TENT ON A LEVEL SURFACE—preferably one that is covered with leaves, pine straw, dirt, or sand—on a tarp or specially designed ground cloth to thwart ground moisture and protect the tent floor. Please avoid pitching a tent in a High Sierra meadow, a particularly fragile and easily damaged environment. Pick up small rocks and sticks that can damage your tent floor and make sleep uncomfortable. Keep a rainfly rolled up at the base of your tent just in case.

- TAKE A SLEEPING PAD WITH YOU. Choose one that is fulllength and thicker than you think you'll need. It will not only keep your hips from aching on hard ground but will also help keep you warm.

- BE WARY OF STANDING DEAD TREES and storm-damaged living trees, which can pose a real hazard to tent campers. These trees may have loose or broken limbs that could fall at any time. When choosing a spot to rest or a backcountry campsite, look up.

Trail and Camping Etiquette

Great care and resources (from nature as well as from your tax dollars) have gone into creating these trails. Treat the trail, wildlife, and fellow hikers with respect.

- **HIKE ON OPEN TRAILS ONLY.**

- **LEAVE ONLY FOOTPRINTS.** Be sensitive to the ground beneath you. Stay on existing trails rather than blazing new ones. Pack out what you pack in.

- **NEVER SPOOK ANIMALS.** An unannounced approach, a sudden movement, or a loud noise startles most animals. Give them extra room and time to adjust to your presence.

- **PLAN AHEAD.** Know your equipment, your ability, and the area where you are hiking—and prepare accordingly. Be self-sufficient at all times; carry necessary supplies for changes in weather or other conditions. A well-executed trip is satisfying.

- **BE COURTEOUS** to other hikers or equestrians you meet on the trails.

- **OBTAIN ALL PERMITS** and authorization as required. Make sure to check in, pay your fee, and mark your site as directed. Don't make the mistake of grabbing a seemingly empty site that looks more appealing than yours—it could be reserved.

- **STRICTLY FOLLOW EACH PARK'S RULES** regarding the building of campfires. It is firmly discouraged and against regulations at most campsites.

N

0   5   10
miles

50
Echo Summit
89
89
88
11
10
9
Markleeville
Round
Top
89
208
395
208
338
NEVADA
CALIFORNIA

MOKELUMNE
WILDERNESS
Highland
Peak
4
8
7
CARSON-ICEBERG
WILDERNESS
Middle
Sister
6

Pacific Crest Trail

Dardanelle
5
4
108
395
182
EMIGRANT
WILDERNESS
HOOVER
WILDERNESS
Bridgeport
108

Tower
Peak
HUMBOLDT-TOIYABE
NATIONAL FOREST
Excelsior
Mtn.
Mono
Lake

Lee Vining
Mt.
Hoffman
120
INYO
NATIONAL
FOREST

3 2
TUOLUMNE
MEADOWS

Pacific Crest Trail

120
Yosemite
Village   YOSEMITE VALLEY
Mt. Lyell
395
YOSEMITE
NATIONAL
PARK
ANSEL ADAMS
WILDERNESS
1
41
Mt. Ritter
203
Mammoth
Lakes

1

SOUTH

Agnew Meadows to
CA Highway 50

1 Agnew Meadows to Thousand Island Lake

SCENERY: ✪ ✪ ✪ ✪ ✪	DISTANCE: *14.8 miles round-trip*
TRAIL CONDITION: ✪ ✪ ✪ ✪ ✪	HIKING TIME: *8–10 hours, or two days*
CHILDREN: ✪ ✪ ✪	MAP: Devils Postpile *by Tom Harrison Maps*
DIFFICULTY: ✪ ✪ ✪	OUTSTANDING FEATURES: *Incredible glaciated*
SOLITUDE: ✪	*mountain views, Thousand Island Lake*

Set in the geologically outstanding Ansel Adams Wilderness, this popular trail offers day hikers and backpackers traveling on the Pacific Crest Trail the opportunity to enjoy sweeping vistas, excellent swimming at Thousand Island Lake, and a number of alpine-lake side trips along the way.

🚶🚶 Starting inside the Devil's Postpile National Monument area (which charges a fee Memorial Day through Labor Day), you'll pick up the trail at Agnew Meadows, about 4 miles before the Devil's Postpile information kiosk and gift shop.

From the first of two Agnew Meadows parking lots, start climbing up on the PCT, which heads north just past the outhouses. You'll ascend approximately 1,300 feet in about 3 miles over sloping fields of mule's ears and some mature aspen groves. At 2.5 miles, you gain an impressive view of Shadow Lake perched hundreds of feet above the Middle Fork of the San Joaquin. The lake is nestled in a glacier-carved pot of granite and backed by the jagged Ritter Range.

From here, the PCT rolls along nicely, climbing slightly less than 300 feet in a little less than 6 miles beneath the 11,000-foot Two Teats and 11,500-foot San Joaquin Mountain on its way to Thousand Island Lake. Overnighters might want to take advantage of a number of side trips along the way. Three different routes to Clark Lakes, a popular destination for anglers, branch off toward the right (north) as the PCT heads in a more northwesterly direction toward

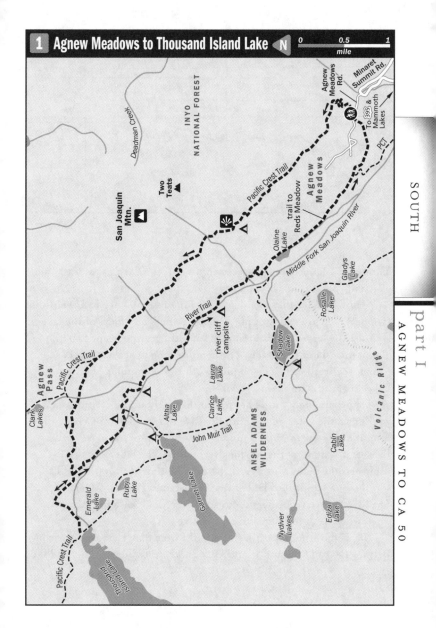

N

0   0.5   1
mile

Minaret Summit Rd.

Agnew Meadows Rd.

To 395 & Mammoth Lakes

PCT

Agnew Meadows

INYO NATIONAL FOREST

Deadman Creek

Two Teats

San Joaquin Mtn.

Pacific Crest Trail

trail to Reds Meadow

Olaine Lake

Middle Fork San Joaquin River

Gladys Lake

Rosalie Lake

River Trail

river cliff campsite

Laura Lake

Clarice Lake

Shadow Lake

Volcanic Ridge

Agnew Pass

Pacific Crest Trail

Clark Lakes

Altha Lake

John Muir Trail

Cabin Lake

ANSEL ADAMS WILDERNESS

Emerald Lake

Ruby Lake

Garnet Lake

Nydiver Lakes

Ediza Lake

Pacific Crest Trail

Thousand Island Lake

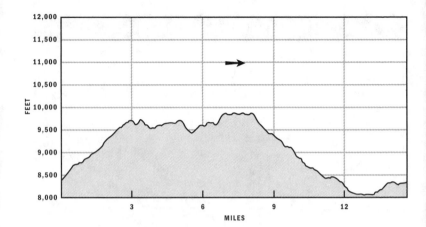

Thousand Island Lake. The second turnoff to Clark Lakes is the most efficient route to reach the lakes.

Thousand Island Lake shares a strong resemblance to Lake Aloha (see page 78) just west of Lake Tahoe on the PCT. Each of the lakes is unusually large and littered with smooth, granite islands. While Thousand Island Lake takes a little more time to access than Lake Aloha, the trailhead, located just north of the popular Mammoth Lakes region, is just as crowded.

Approximately 1 mile before reaching Thousand Island Lake, you'll pass the intersection with the River Trail. Upon reaching the lake, it's obvious that the opportunities for exploration are endless. In fact, it is here, at the northeastern end of the lake, that the PCT intersects the John Muir Trail. If you have time, follow the JMT south past a handful of lakes, including Emerald, Ruby, Garnet, and Shadow, before reconnecting to the River Trail for a beautiful and worthwhile 4-mile extension to this hike.

Backed by the impressively rugged Ritter Range, most noticeably Banner Peak, Thousand Island Lake is the headwaters of the Middle

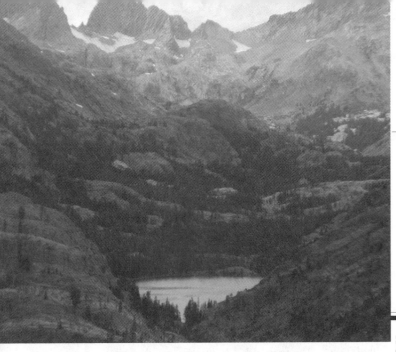

Gain incredible views of Shadow Lake and the Ritter Range from the PCT on the way to Thousand Island Lake.

Fork of the San Joaquin River, a watershed that rushes freely in the springtime and barely trickles after summer's gone.

Follow the river's path on the River Trail as it descends back to Agnew Meadows through dense pine-and-hardwood forest. Along the way, you'll find a couple of backpacker campsites along the riverbank and trails leading to Garnet and Shadow lakes.

Exactly 1 mile after turning south onto the River Trail from the PCT, there is an unmarked trail that branches off to the right (southwest); follow this trail approximately 0.5 miles to reach Garnet Lake, an incredibly scenic lake with great camping around its shoreline. Approximately 3 miles downstream, a trail leading 1.9 miles up to Shadow Lake (marked) also branches off to the right (west). Camping is also available at Shadow Lake along the creek at its west end, but is prohibited around the lake.

The last mile of this loop hike can be confusing to follow. At the first sign and trail junction after the trail to Shadow Lake is a trail that continues to Reds Meadow. Stay to the left (traveling southeast) and continue to Agnew Meadows. Approximately 0.5 miles after the sign to Reds Meadow there is a sign that directs traffic to Agnew Meadows. Keep right at this sign to avoid returning through horse-filled campgrounds.

DIRECTIONS Exit US 395 to Mammoth Junction 26 miles south of Lee Vining. Turn west on CA 203/Minaret Summit Road and drive 14 miles to the Agnew Meadows Campground. There is an entrance fee Memorial Day through Labor Day.

If you're visiting mid-June through mid-September, there is a mandatory shuttle departing from the Mammoth Mountain Ski Area Gondola Building adjacent to the Mammoth Mountain Inn at the top of CA 203. Due to the volume of traffic, private vehicles are not allowed into the monument area. At the time of publication, round-trip shuttle fees were $7 for adults, $4 for children, and $20 per carload. Call the Mammoth Lakes Visitor Center at (760) 924-5500 for details.

PERMITS Overnight backpackers must obtain a backcountry permit; reserve in advance by calling (760) 873-2483 or pick up a walk-in permit at the Mammoth Lakes Visitor Center, located at 2520 Main Street in Mammoth Lakes, starting at 11 a.m. the day before your trip starts. More information is available at www.nps.gov/depo.

GPS Trailhead Coordinates	1 Agnew Meadows to Thousand Island Lake
UTM Zone (WGS 84)	11S
Easting	0316187
Northing	4172670
Latitude	N37° 40.9700'
Longitude	W119° 5.0722'

2 Tuolumne Meadows
to Ireland Lake

SCENERY: ✿ ✿ ✿ ✿ ✿	HIKING TIME: *Overnight*
TRAIL CONDITION: ✿ ✿ ✿ ✿ ✿	MAP: Yosemite High Country *by Tom*
CHILDREN: ✿ ✿	*Harrison Maps*
DIFFICULTY: ✿ ✿ ✿ ✿	OUTSTANDING FEATURES: *Ireland Lake,*
SOLITUDE: ✿ ✿	*Vogelsang High Sierra Camp, wildflowers,*
DISTANCE: *22.3 miles round-trip*	*Lyell Canyon*

There's a reason Yosemite is one of the nation's most visited national parks. Yosemite's high country, although less dramatic than its valley, does not disappoint. This beautiful overnight journey features a night out at Ireland Lake and is a must-see for outdoor photographers; the sunsets here last for hours.

🚶🚶 The Pacific Crest Trail cuts right through Tuolumne Meadows as it follows Lyell Canyon. Pick up the trail at the Dog Lake parking lot past the Tuolumne Meadows Ranger Station. Before you go, you'll need to invest in a bear canister if you want to be legal and keep the food you packed in safe. Canisters are $5 for up to two weeks with a $65 deposit refunded upon return.

You'll also need a free permit to camp in the backcountry (see page 30 for details). Permits are most easily obtained at the ranger station in person on the day of your hike. Permits to Vogelsang fill up less quickly than permits to some of the other Yosemite backcountry destinations, but it's still a good idea to head into the ranger station early. They open at 8 a.m.

For this hike, you'll need to consider your hiking style. I prefer to tackle short, steep climbs rather than short, steep descents. My lungs are healthy and my calves are strong enough to handle a steep climb, but my knees don't fare as well on a steep descent, especially loaded with a pack. Plus I'd rather put my mind to a climb and finish it quickly than settle in for a long, steady ascent.

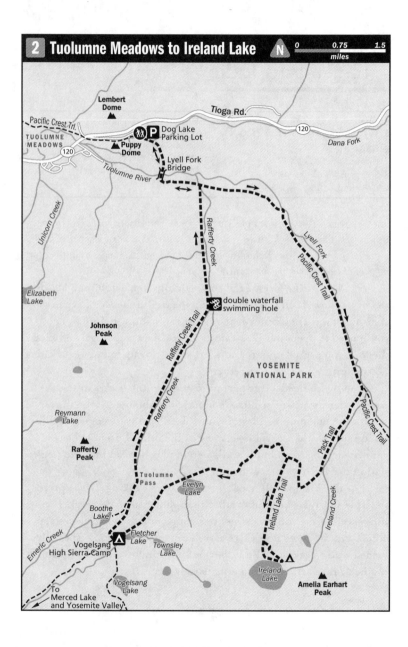

Lembert
Dome

Tioga Rd.

Pacific Crest Trl.

120

TUOLUMNE
MEADOWS

Dana Fork

120

Dog Lake
Parking Lot

Puppy
Dome

Tuolumne River

Lyell Fork
Bridge

Unicorn Creek

Rafferty Creek

Lyell Fork

Pacific Crest Trail

Elizabeth
Lake

double waterfall
swimming hole

Johnson
Peak

Rafferty Creek Trail

YOSEMITE
NATIONAL PARK

Reymann
Lake

Rafferty Creek

Rafferty
Peak

Pack Trail

Tuolumne
Pass

Evelyn
Lake

Pacific Crest Trail

Boothe
Lake

Ireland Lake Trail

Fletcher
Lake

Ireland Creek

Emeric Creek

Vogelsang
High Sierra Camp

Townsley
Lake

Vogelsang
Lake

To
Merced Lake
and Yosemite Valley

Ireland
Lake

Amelia Earhart
Peak

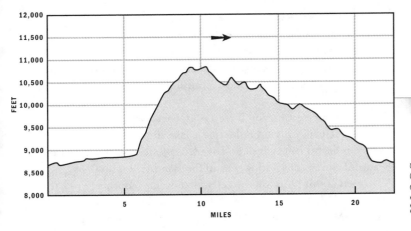

These preferences made me decide to tackle this hike in a clock-wise direction, but many folks opt to hike a counterclockwise loop. You can decide for yourself what's best for you. Clockwise, you'll climb from 8,800 feet to 10,425 (1,625 feet) in 2.6 miles and will descend the same elevation over a course of 12.6 miles. Counterclockwise, you'll climb 1,625 feet over a course of 12.6 miles and will then steeply descend 2.6 miles before finishing along the relatively flat terrain through Lyell Canyon. If you can handle a steep climb, the clockwise loop takes less time and descends more gradually. My description fol-lows the clockwise loop.

From the trailhead, follow the combination PCT and John Muir Trail, which heads east and southeast along the peaceful Lyell River Canyon. After 1.6 miles you see a junction with the Rafferty Creek Trail branching off to the right (due south). This is the most direct route to Vogelsang High Sierra Camp, and it is also the trail you'll return on for the clockwise loop hike. For now, follow the PCT another 3.8 miles to the intersection with the pack trail to Vogelsang.

The PCT follows Lyell Canyon just out of view of the actual river for much of this distance. However, there are some nice swimming and fishing holes along the way and I recommend taking your time through the canyon. The climb up the pack trail to the intersection of the Ireland Lake Trail follows a steep grade through dense forest.

At the intersection you'll see a sign that says 3 miles to Ireland Lake. It's actually only 1.5 miles to the lake after this junction, gaining around 400 feet to Ireland Lake (10,750 feet) as you pass through beautiful clumps of wildflowers and thousands of mosquitoes.

It was at this point on one very memorable scouting trip that I, already hobbled by a throbbing blister on my heel, developed early stages of Mosquito Anxiety Disorder, or MAD. It's amazing how quickly this condition can advance, so treat the symptoms early. Reapply bug spray, change into a long-sleeved shirt and pants, put on your bug net, take a deep breath, and most importantly, calmly announce that you're suffering from MAD and have the potential to behave irrationally.

If you treat your MAD early, you will thoroughly enjoy coming upon Ireland Lake. The last steps to the lake crest an emerald-green rolling lawn. While Ireland Lake was named after Dr. Merritte Weber Ireland (who was stationed in Yosemite in the late nineteenth century), it's not hard to imagine you've dropped down the proverbial rabbit hole and are suddenly in the land of Ireland upon reaching this lake.

The best camping is on a flat perch (much of the ground is lumpy from marmot hole construction) on the east side of the lake near Ireland Creek. Settle in and watch the reflection of Amelia Earhart Peak in Ireland Lake and alpenglow that goes forever as the sun slowly sinks behind the Cathedral Range. This is an excellent opportunity for photographers to catch fantastic lighting over the lake and surrounding meadows.

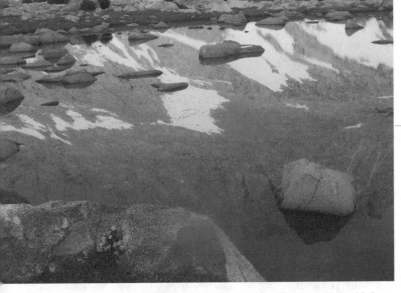

Catch the alpenglow on Amelia Earhart Peak reflected in the still waters of Ireland Lake.

From Ireland Lake, it's 14 miles back to your starting point but well worth it. To complete the loop, follow the trail to Vogelsang High Sierra Camp, approximately 3.5 miles through bucolic meadows and past a couple of unnamed lakes plus picturesque Evelyn Lake and finally Fletcher Lake. If you arrive between 1 and 5 p.m. at Vogelsang High Sierra Camp, the store should be open. Just outside of the camp you'll come to a four-way intersection; from here the options are endless. You could follow a loop trail to Merced Lake, passing Babcock Lake, Emery Lake, Burmese Lake, and Vogelsang Pass along the way.

However, for this hike and in the interest of a simple weekend trip, continue to Lyell Canyon, following Rafferty Creek loosely as the trail descends to Tuolumne Meadows. The first turnoff you pass after leaving Vogelsang leads to Boothe Lake, a 1-mile side trip worthwhile for the swimming.

The other point of interest is a double waterfall into a pool on Rafferty Creek that lies just out of sight from the trail. Many people will walk right past the noise of rushing water, but if you hear it, follow it and your reward will be a cool pool at the bottom of two small waterfalls plunging side by side.

Upon reaching the PCT again, turn left to return to the parking lot.

DIRECTIONS   From CA 395 follow CA 120 (Tioga Pass Rd.) west for 18.6 miles. Turn left on Tuolumne Lodge Road and follow it 0.4 miles. Turn left into the Dog Lake parking lot.

From the west, travel east on CA 120 (Tioga Road) for 40 miles from the Big Oak Flat Entrance Station, before reaching the right turn onto Tuolumne Lodge Road, just past the Tuolumne Meadows Grill.

PERMITS AND FEES   All vehicles entering Yosemite National Park must pay a $20 entrance fee or present either a Yosemite Pass ($40) or an America the Beautiful annual pass ($80). Free wilderness permits are required year-round for overnight trips only and can be obtained in person at the Tuolumne Meadows Ranger Station the morning of your hike. Reservations can be made up to 24 weeks in advance for a fee; visit www.nps.gov/yose/planyourvisitwildpermits.htm for details.

GPS Trailhead Coordinates   2 Tuolumne Meadows to
Ireland Lake
UTM Zone (WGS 84)   11S
Easting   0294330
Northing   4194826
Latitude   N37° 52.6636'
Longitude   W119° 20.3110'

3 Tuolumne Meadows to Waterwheel Falls

SCENERY: ✿ ✿ ✿ ✿ ✿	HIKING TIME: *Overnight*
TRAIL CONDITION: ✿ ✿ ✿ ✿ ✿	MAP: Yosemite High Country *by Tom*
CHILDREN: ✿ ✿ ✿ ✿	*Harrison Maps*
DIFFICULTY: ✿ ✿	OUTSTANDING FEATURES: *Tuolumne*
SOLITUDE: ✿	*Meadows, wildflowers, waterfalls (LeConte,*
DISTANCE: *16 miles round-trip*	*California, Tuolumne, and Waterwheel)*

In the words of John Muir, you just might feel as though "this is the most spacious and delightful high pleasure ground" you've yet to see. The well-traveled Pacific Crest Trail through Tuolumne Meadows and into Glen Aulin reveals a lively river with dozens of cascades and clear emerald pools and in midsummer is lush with wildflowers.

🚶🚶 Unless you're traveling to Waterwheel Falls in winter, you won't have trouble figuring out how to get there. The trails are more than adequately signed the whole way, and the amount of foot traffic in the area is about quadruple of that elsewhere on the PCT. There's a good reason—the scenic beauty from the very first step to the last.

Before you start, make sure to pick up a permit for wilderness travel at the Tuolumne Meadows Ranger Station. A permit to Glen Aulin can be picked up on the same day of travel—just try to make it in early before all the permits are gone. Weekends fill up fast, so consider making a reservation (see page 35 for details).

Starting from the Soda Springs/Glen Aulin Trailhead, park alongside the road and immediately empty the car of anything fragrant, as black bears in this area are an opportunistic bunch who thrive on the tourist industry. Stow your smelly stuff—any food, gum, wine, sunscreen, tea—in one of the dozens of bear lockers and make note of the number (they all look the same). You'll also need a bear canister to store any food you might pack in.

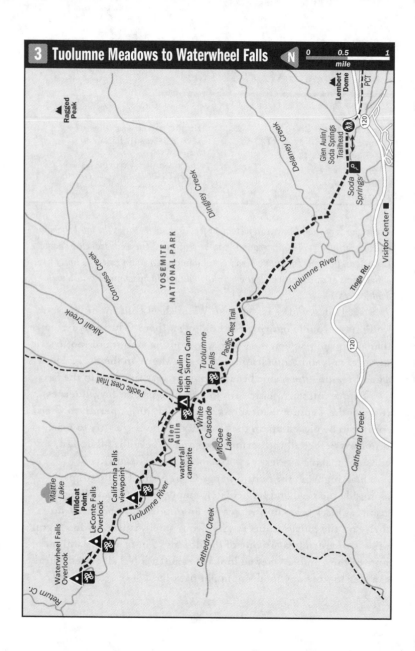

N

0   0.5   1
mile

Lembert Dome

PCT

Ragged Peak

Delaney Creek

Glen Aulin/ Soda Springs Trailhead

120

Soda Springs

Visitor Center

Dingley Creek

Tioga Rd.

YOSEMITE NATIONAL PARK

Conness Creek

Tuolumne River

Pacific Crest Trail

Alkali Creek

Pacific Crest Trail

Glen Aulin High Sierra Camp

Tuolumne Falls

120

White Cascade

Glen Aulin

McGee Lake

Cathedral Creek

waterfall campsite

Mattie Lake

Wildcat Point

California Falls viewpoint

LeConte Falls Overlook

Tuolumne River

Cathedral Creek

Waterwheel Falls Overlook

Return Cr.

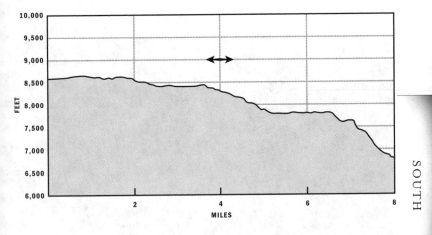

Once you start hiking, views of the placid Tuolumne River meandering through the meadow with a host of outstanding peaks in the distance make excellent picture opportunities. If you can stop taking pictures long enough to hike, you'll find the beginnings of an interpretive trail. The PCT follows the trail for a few signs, but if you want to continue to Glen Aulin, veer away from the river and continue on the PCT heading north.

After 3.8 miles you come to the first prominent cascade on the Tuolumne, seen right off the trail, Tuolumne Falls. In approximately another mile there's a major intersection with a trail leading to McGee Lake, part of the high-country camp route that many hikers travel, starting with Glen Aulin High Sierra Camp, which is about 0.25 miles down the hill. It sits off the trail at the base of White Cascade and above another unnamed waterfall and is a great overnight option for families or folks who are looking for home-cooked meals, a nice flat bed, and the community of other campers.

Glen Aulin fills up. In fact, I've been issued the very last permit to travel into Glen Aulin at 9 a.m. in the middle of July. Renting

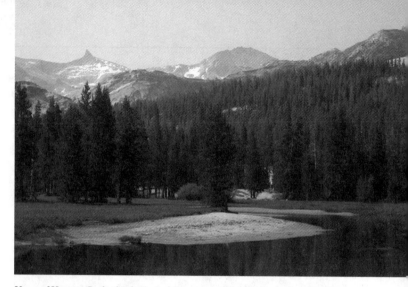

Views of Unicorn Peak, the Cathedral Range, and Fairview Dome from Tuolumne Meadows will take your breath away on the way to Waterwheel Falls.

a tent cabin for the night at Glen Aulin High Sierra Camp (which includes breakfast and dinner) isn't cheap, but it does save on the weight you'll carry in. Regardless, it's a good place to use a proper restroom and fill up on filtered water before traveling down canyon.

For a more remote wilderness camping experience, veer left off the PCT and into the Grand Canyon of the Tuolumne. It's all downhill from here. First you'll enter Glen Aulin, the meadows famous for their hip-high lupines. Swaths of purple line the trail as far as the eye can see.

Campsites are few and far between before reaching California Falls, but I have found a site that's worth sharing (and tempting to keep secret). After 6 miles from the start, wander off the trail and over to the river (you can hear it from the trail); there, on top of a smooth granite slope are a few good sites fit for two people. The site sits right above a waterfall, and the sunset and sunrise views are dramatic.

Stash your camping gear and head downstream to check off more waterfall sightings. California Falls is probably the most impressive as far as the viewpoint goes, and it is approximately 0.5 miles from the waterfall campsite. The trail drops steeply into the canyon, and in another 0.5 miles there's an overlook of the dramatic, spitting rooster tail at the top of LeConte Falls.

Approximately 0.5 miles downstream of LeConte is the top of Waterwheel Falls, a cascade that seems to drop forever into the canyon below. Near the top a spur trail leads to an impressive vista when the water is high (before mid-July in most years). The cascade calms where Return Creek feeds into the Tuolumne River another 0.5 miles downstream, where a footbridge signifies this end.

While the footbridge seems like an obvious destination and turnaround point, it's no more scenic than the top of the falls and getting there requires a very steep descent and ascent.

DIRECTIONS Traveling west on CA 120 (Tioga Road), turn right into the Soda Springs/Glen Aulin Trailhead.

PERMITS AND FEES All vehicles entering Yosemite National Park must pay a $20 entrance fee or present either a Yosemite Pass ($40) or an America the Beautiful annual pass ($80). Free wilderness permits are required year-round for overnight trips only and can be obtained in person at the Tuolumne Meadows Ranger Station the morning of your hike. Be aware that quotas can fill up quickly on busy weekends. Reservations can be made up to 24 weeks in advance for a fee; visit www.nps.gov/yose/planyourvisitwildpermits.htm for details.

GPS Trailhead Coordinates	3 Tuolumne Meadows to Waterwheel Falls
UTM Zone (WGS 84)	11S
Easting	0292585
Northing	4195010
Latitude	N37° 52.7390′
Longitude	W119° 21.5035′

4 Sonora Pass to Leavitt Lake

SCENERY: ✿ ✿ ✿ ✿ ✿
TRAIL CONDITION: ✿ ✿ ✿
CHILDREN: ✿ (✿ ✿ *if overnight*)
DIFFICULTY: ✿ ✿ ✿ ✿ ✿
SOLITUDE: ✿ ✿
DISTANCE: *16 miles round-trip*

HIKING TIME: *8–12 hours, or 2 days*
MAP: Emigrant Wilderness *by Tom Harrison Maps*
OUTSTANDING FEATURES: *High mountain views, alpine lakes, wildlife, Leavitt Lake*

An ambitious day hike with nonstop panoramic views, this 16-mile-round-trip High Sierra loop follows the scenic back side of a few 10,000-plus-foot peaks with four great fishing lakes lying in their shadows. Explore them at lake level or satisfy yourself with the view—either way, this hike is a Pacific Crest Trail classic with a taste of off-trail adventure.

🏃 Begin this hike at the road sign that reads SONORA PASS on the south side of CA 108. From the beginning, there's a clear view of what's ahead. The trail climbs rapidly from the start and then follows the midline of a broad mountain bowl before stepping onto the ridgeline you'll follow for most of the way. Because most of the hike is above tree line, the view of the trail is as clear as the views of distant mountain peaks, so it's pretty easy to walk and let the views sink in.

After following the ridgeline and scree fields immediately beneath the ridges, the trail drops into a notch. Here, you'll see the four lakes: Latopie, the closest; then Upper and Lower Koenig lakes; and farthest away, Leavitt Lake.

A faintly traveled trail heads directly to Latopie Lake, a small, clear lake. This short but steep side trip could be a mere detour to cool the skin on a hot summer day, before returning to the PCT and continuing the ridge hike south to Leavitt Lake. Or you could do what the locals do: Follow the drainage to the north of Latopie Lake down to the Koenig lakes and Leavitt Lake and make a loop hike.

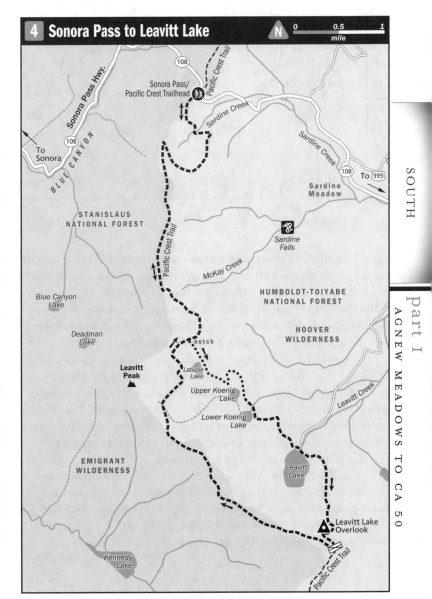

N

0   0.5   1
mile

108

Sonora Pass/
Pacific Crest Trailhead

Pacific Crest Trail

Sardine Creek

Sardine Creek

108

To 395

Sonora Pass Hwy.

108

To
Sonora

BLUE CANYON

Sardine
Meadow

STANISLAUS
NATIONAL FOREST

Sardine
Falls

Pacific Crest Trail

McKay Creek

HUMBOLDT-TOIYABE
NATIONAL FOREST

Blue Canyon
Lake

HOOVER
WILDERNESS

Deadman
Lake

notch

Leavitt
Peak

Latopie
Lake

Leavitt Creek

Upper Koenig
Lake

Lower Koenig
Lake

EMIGRANT
WILDERNESS

Leavitt
Lake

Leavitt Lake
Overlook

Kennedy
Lake

Pacific Crest Trail

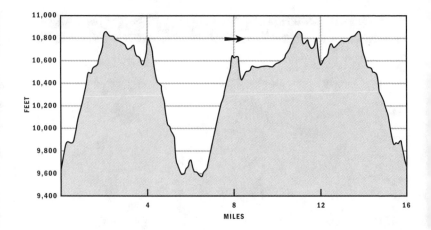

The trail, faint at best and invisible at worst, follows the drainage (or dry creek bed) and after some slippery, steep spots connects with the marshy Koenig lakes. Although this trail is anything but regularly maintained, three key things will keep you on the right track: First, follow the drainage; second, don't go below 9,500 feet in elevation; and third, keep right as you drop into the meadow.

A two-track road leads to Upper Koenig Lake from the north. Cross the road and a marshy stream that empties into the emerald lake and come to Lower Koenig Lake, a small but deep lake that's good for swimming (though you won't find a real beach). Take a quick dip or simply soak your feet before hooking up with a trail that goes around Lower Koenig Lake and leads to Leavitt Lake, a very popular fishing lake accessed by a 4WD road.

From Leavitt Lake, head south to climb onto the ridgeline and find the PCT again. There's a maze of dirt roads and it's easy to get disoriented. Keep right on the first double-wide track and when the roads split into three forks, take the middle path for the most direct route to the PCT. The trail climbs steeply and steadily to the

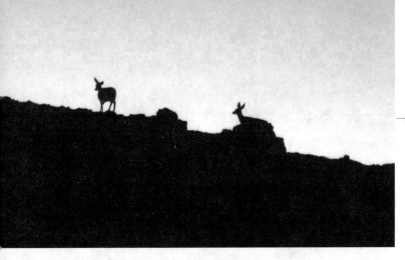

Some mule deer spend the summer in the high country above Sonora Pass.

southeast of Leavitt Lake before coming to a T. A right turn leads to
an amazing overlook of Leavitt Lake—probably the most scenic spot
on the trail and a nice place to rest after the solid climbing. Turn
around and follow the trail to the south (left from the T) to reach the
10,660-foot crest as you go through a gated area. Amazing views of
Yosemite open up to the south.

Keep right, or northwest, on the PCT to complete the loop. The
trail winds along the back of exposed lava-scree slope with a sustained
drop-off and partial views of Deadman Lake and Blue Canyon Lake
nearly 3,000 feet below. Dozens of peaks and foothill canyons frame
the skyline as you complete the circuit. Winds often howl over this
ridgeline return route, so pack a windproof layer any time of year.

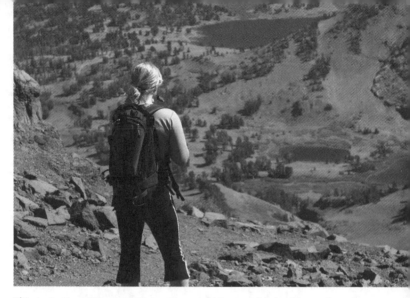

Take in the view of Upper and Lower Koenig and Leavitt lakes from the notch.

DIRECTIONS   Sonora Pass is 14.7 miles west of the CA 395/108 junction. Trailhead parking is 0.2 miles west of the pass. The trail starts on the south side of CA 108 at the pass signage.

PERMITS   Free wilderness permits are required for overnight trips in the both Emigrant Wilderness (generally west of the PCT) and Hoover Wilderness (generally east of the PCT). Reservations are not necessary. Hikers can pick up permits at the Summit Ranger District if coming from the west or the Bridgeport Ranger District if coming from the east (see page 175 for contact information). Hikers need to be aware of campfire regulations, which change throughout the season.

GPS Trailhead Coordinates	4 Sonora Pass to Leavitt Lake
UTM Zone (WGS 84)	11S
Easting	269832
Northing	4243284
Latitude	N38° 30.8130′
Longitude	W119° 63.2420′

5 Sonora Pass to Sonora Peak

SCENERY: ✿ ✿ ✿ ✿ ✿	HIKING TIME: *3–5 hours*
TRAIL CONDITION: ✿ ✿ ✿	MAP: Emigrant Wilderness *by Tom*
CHILDREN: ✿ ✿	*Harrison Maps*
DIFFICULTY: ✿ ✿ ✿	OUTSTANDING FEATURES: *Windswept vistas,*
SOLITUDE: ✿ ✿	*wildflowers in early to midsummer, volcanic geology*
DISTANCE: *7 miles round-trip*	

Bagging Sonora Peak is as close as you can get to flying without your feet leaving the ground. This rewarding summit provides nonstop spectacular views start to finish. The only problem with this hike at all is that at some point you'll have to leave the summit.

🚶🚶 Although the views take the breath away with every step, it's easy to see why the U.S. Marine Corps has a mountain warfare training camp at the base of Sonora Pass just 4 miles from the CA 108 junction with US 395. This is a harsh environment. Even on a nice day, expect high winds that have the power to chill to the bone. Keep that in mind if the notion of dragging junior to Sonora Peak (elevation 11,500 feet) strikes—this is a hike for children of the very hearty variety.

The trail begins climbing from the start and doesn't let up much until the top. Very few trees provide shade, which is great for the vistas but leaves the wind free to howl and gives the sun a direct shot at your face—be prepared with extra layers and sunscreen.

Sage, mule's ears, and colorful wildflowers midsummer make the hillside sparkle against the purple-red volcanic ground and rocks. Birds are plentiful along the multiple lush streambeds that trickle down the mountain and across the trail. This is a good hike to bring the binoculars, with vistas stretching for miles. Along the way there is one somewhat developed campsite; a good spot to watch a meteor shower.

As you ascend, you'll notice a prominent, bulbous collection of volcanic spires. The spires are an interesting place to explore, with a

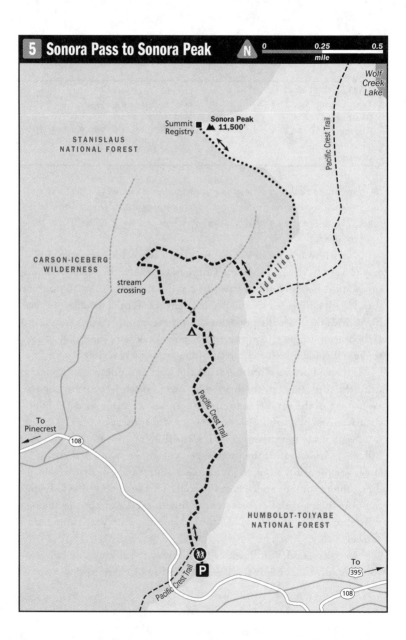

N

0   0.25   0.5
mile

Wolf
Creek
Lake

Pacific Crest Trail

Summit
Registry

Sonora Peak
▲ 11,500'

STANISLAUS
NATIONAL FOREST

CARSON-ICEBERG
WILDERNESS

stream
crossing

ridgeline

Pacific Crest Trail

To
Pinecrest

108

HUMBOLDT-TOIYABE
NATIONAL FOREST

To
395

Pacific Crest Trail

108

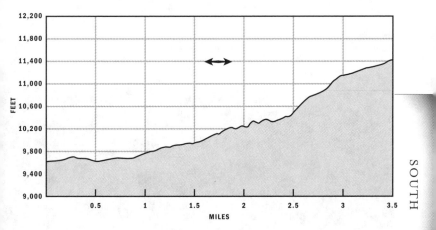

few caves and natural arches, but few hikers make the detour, probably due to the slippery volcanic scree that guards the feature.

The PCT winds up to the top of the spires, and that's exactly where you'll find the faint trail leading the rest of the way to Sonora Peak, up and to the left. From this junction it's a little more than 1.2 miles of climbing to the summit.

The spur trail is pretty easy to follow, but it also disappears in a few places. My advice is to keep your head up and avoid traveling at night if it's your first time to the peak (even on my descent I found the trail to be more difficult to follow).

Making the summit is an indescribable feeling, although scores of previous hikers have tried to depict it in the summit register stashed in the highest of three rock-built wind shelters. The description I found most amusing was one that called the hike "an ovary buster but well worth it." Being at the summit makes you feel like a bird. Clouds race overhead, dappling the landscape for miles, forming and reforming like giant jellyfish in the sky. In the words of an

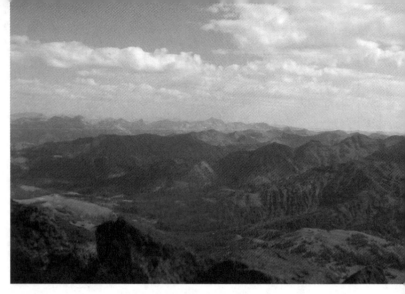

Southern views from Sonora Peak (11,500 feet) stretch into Yosemite National Park.

anonymous registry entry, "It's time to roam the mountains and set the spirit free."

DIRECTIONS From the intersection of CA 108 with US 395, travel west on CA 108 to Sonora Pass (elevation 9,624 feet). The trailhead and parking area are 200 yards past the summit on the right.

PERMITS Free wilderness permits are required for overnight trips in Carson-Iceberg Wilderness and can be obtained in person at the Summit Ranger District. See page 175 for contact information.

GPS Trailhead Coordinates	5 Sonora Pass to Sonora Peak
UTM Zone (WGS 84)	11S
Easting	0269651
Northing	4245692
Latitude	N38° 19.7866′
Longitude	W119° 38.1162′

6 Clark Fork to Disaster Creek

SCENERY: ✿ ✿ ✿ ✿ ✿	DISTANCE: *15 miles round-trip*
TRAIL CONDITION: ✿ ✿ ✿	HIKING TIME: *8 hours or overnight*
CHILDREN: ✿	MAP: *USFS* A Guide to the Carson-
DIFFICULTY: ✿ ✿ ✿ ✿ ✿	Iceberg Wilderness
SOLITUDE: ✿ ✿ ✿ ✿ ✿	OUTSTANDING FEATURES: *Mountain vistas,*
	Boulder Lake, scenic Disaster Creek

Explore the Carson-Iceberg Wilderness along the Clark Fork, Pacific Crest, and Disaster Creek trails. This 15-mile loop hike makes for an ambitious day hike or a spectacular overnight trip, with camping options available at small lakes along the PCT or early on at Boulder Lake.

🚶🚶 Through my research for this book, I've talked with many passionate hikers about routes along the PCT. Kate Reid, owner of San Francisco—based women's backpacking adventure operator Call of the Wild, recommended this route for its incredible scenery, amazing solitude, and high sense of adventure. After scouting it, I agree with her.

Starting from the Clark Fork Trailhead at around 6,500 feet, expect to begin climbing straight away though only moderately so. Over the course of the first 1.5 miles you gain about 400 feet before reaching a trail junction where both trails (heading right and left) continue uphill.

Follow Boulder Creek to the north (left). The trail to Boulder Lake is fairly steep, gaining approximately 1,200 feet in just a little more than 1 mile. The climb is worth it. Boulder Lake is set in a spectacular granite bowl and makes for an excellent spot to wash off the sweat you broke to get to this point. Take advantage of this reliable water source until late in the season and fill up on water for the rest of the journey.

Hook around the northeast side of the lake to reach the PCT approximately 0.75 miles away. Once you reach the PCT (at around

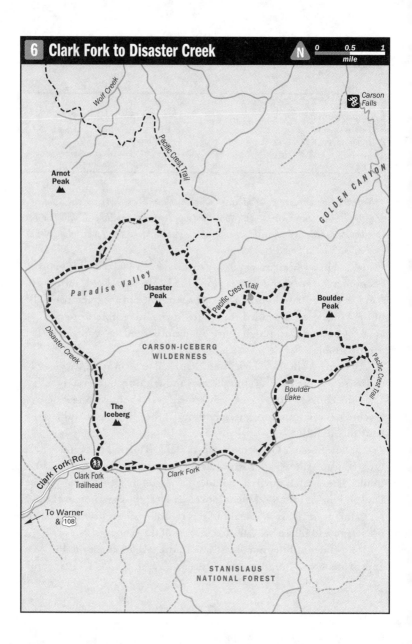

N

0   0.5   1
mile

Wolf Creek

Carson
Falls

Arnot
Peak
▲

Pacific Crest Trail

GOLDEN CANYON

Paradise Valley

Disaster
Peak
▲

Pacific Crest Trail

Boulder
Peak
▲

Disaster Creek

CARSON-ICEBERG
WILDERNESS

Boulder
Lake

Pacific Crest Trail

The
Iceberg
▲

Clark Fork Rd.

Clark Fork
Trailhead

Clark Fork

To Warner
& 108

STANISLAUS
NATIONAL FOREST

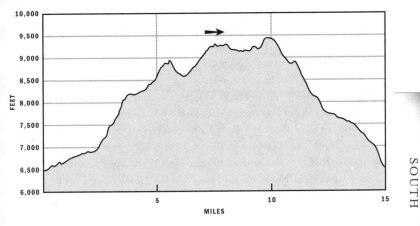

8,500 feet), you are faced with wide open mountain vistas in all directions for the next 4.6 miles.

Enjoy the view as the PCT undulates along the crest, gaining about 1,000 feet before reaching the junction to Paradise Valley. Approximately halfway to this intersection (2.8 miles from the Clark Fork Trail and PCT intersection) there's an excellent option for camping, or for that second snack break, at an unnamed lake on the PCT. Such lakeside camping with all the views is a rare opportunity, and overnighters should take advantage of this location.

After 4.6 miles of hiking on the PCT, you come to a four-way intersection with an unreliably marked trail heading east–west. Turn left (west) here to continue into Paradise Valley. The trail heads straight up a short, steep hill, while the PCT starts to descend.

You reach the top of this hill in very short order, in 400 feet or so, over the course of about 0.25 miles of climbing. Top out on a forested saddle, and the next ridge of mountains will come into view. Thick manzanita bushes line each side of the trail, overgrowing at some points. Shortly after crossing this ridge, you reach the start of a stream. The trail descends steeply—1,200 feet in just more than 2 miles—along the stream. Expect to see plenty of evidence that deer and bears inhabit this rarely visited wilderness area.

After 2 miles of steady descent you reach the junction of Disaster Creek Trail, which runs northwest–southeast from Iceberg Meadow to Highland Lakes. Follow the trail left (southeast) to descend the remaining 2.5 miles along scenic Disaster Creek all the way back to the Clark Fork Trailhead. You'll know you're getting close to the Disaster Creek Trailhead when the trail turns into a series of steep granite switchbacks. From the Disaster Creek Trailhead, follow the gigantic signs a few hundred yards back to the Clark Fork Trailhead.

DIRECTIONS Traveling east on CA 108, turn left onto Clark Fork Road at Wagner (this road may be closed early season due to snowpack). Follow the road until it ends at the Clark Fork Trailhead. Traveling west on CA 108, Clark Ford Road will be on the right, west of Dardanelle and approximately 30 miles from the intersection with US 395.

PERMITS Free wilderness permits are required for overnight trips in Carson-Iceberg Wilderness and can be obtained at the Calaveras and Summit Ranger Stations. Reservations are not necessary. See page 175 for contact information.

GPS Trailhead Coordinates	6 Clark Fork to Disaster Creek
UTM Zone (WGS 84)	11S
Easting	0259955
Northing	4255481
Latitude	N38° 25.0329'
Longitude	W119° 44.9650'

7 Wolf Creek

SCENERY: ☆☆☆	HIKING TIME: *7–9 hours*
TRAIL CONDITION: ☆☆	MAP: *USFS* A Guide to the Carson-Iceberg Wilderness
CHILDREN: ☆☆	OUTSTANDING FEATURES: *Waterfalls and swimming holes on Wolf Creek, sweeping mountain vistas, Asa Lake*
DIFFICULTY: ☆☆☆☆	
SOLITUDE: ☆☆☆	
DISTANCE: *13 miles round-trip*	

The Carson-Iceberg Wilderness south of Ebbetts Pass is a rugged landscape. Giant volcanic peaks, deep-green conifer forest, and handfuls of aspen trees provide a striking palette. In summer, the highlight of this loop hike is the two unnamed, unmarked waterfalls on Wolf Creek and their emerald-clear cascade pools.

In 1853, Major John Ebbett reckoned the route over Ebbetts Pass had "great promise" as "probably the best site for a transcontinental railway." Although that never came to pass, in 1864 merchants in the Gold Rush–town of Murphys (to the west) got together to build the Big Trees to Carson Valley Road (what is now CA 4) to connect with the silver-boom towns on the eastern side of the Sierra. In the 1960s, the road was finally paved in its entirety and adopted into the California highway system.

The native Washoe and Miwok tribes inhabiting the region in summer dwindled following the discovery of gold and silver and the increase in European settlers. The large meadows and streambeds became prime cattle-grazing lands. Summer cattle-grazing remains a prominent feature of this landscape today, as permitted by the Wilderness Act of 1964, and amended in 1984 to add the Carson-Iceberg Wilderness.

You're just as likely to hear the chorus of cowbells as the screech of a hawk soaring overhead. Between 200 and 300 wildlife species make this wilderness their home. On your hike, you might get a good glimpse of some of these rare species—the Lahontan cutthroat trout

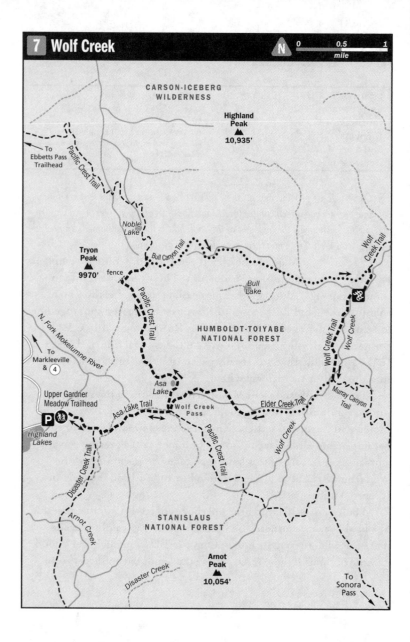

N

0   0.5   1
mile

CARSON-ICEBERG
WILDERNESS

Highland
Peak
10,935'

To
Ebbetts Pass
Trailhead

Pacific Crest Trail

Noble
Lake

Bull Canyon Trail

Tryon
Peak
9970'   fence

Pacific Crest Trail

Bull
Lake

Wolf Creek Trail

HUMBOLDT-TOIYABE
NATIONAL FOREST

N. Fork Mokelumne River

To
Markleeville
& 4

Wolf Creek Trail

Wolf Creek

Upper Gardner
Meadow Trailhead

P

Asa Lake Trail

Asa
Lake

Wolf Creek
Pass

Elder Creek Trail

Murray Canyon
Trail

Highland
Lakes

Disaster Creek Trail

Pacific Crest Trail

Wolf Creek

Arnot Creek

STANISLAUS
NATIONAL FOREST

Disaster Creek

Arnot
Peak
10,054'

To
Sonora
Pass

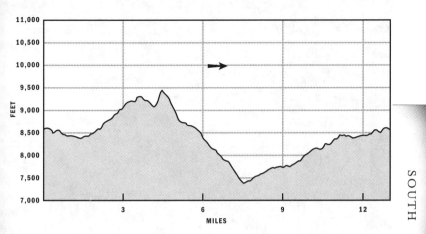

and Paiute cutthroat trout, for instance. Or you just might see herds of wild cow. Either way, this 13-mile loop hike is an adventure.

The hike begins at the Upper Gardner Meadow Trailhead in Stanislaus National Forest east of Highland Lakes. After entering the Carson-Iceberg Wilderness at 0.5 miles there is a sign and fork in the trail. Right (south) heads to Disaster Creek, while left (north) continues 1.3 miles to the intersection with the Pacific Crest Trail leading to Asa Lake. Continue toward Asa Lake (small enough that it's unmarked on many maps). Follow the PCT north around the east side of Asa Lake. Asa Lake is small but very pretty, and it doesn't take long to stop off at the lake and resume hiking on the PCT, which follows a few switchbacks above the lake to the pass below Tryon Peak.

The hike to Asa Lake is a popular day hike since the 2.5-mile one-way distance has very little gradient change. It's also a good hike for families with children.

For those continuing north, the PCT climbs before traversing the windy ridge south of Tryon Peak and provides excellent views to Highland Lakes and into the 161,181-acre Carson-Iceberg

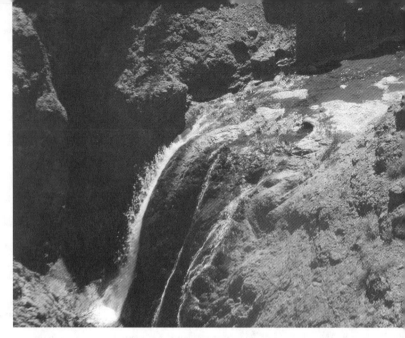

Two (unnamed) cascades on Wolf Creek pour over volcanic rock and into deep pools.

Wilderness. At 3.5 miles from the Upper Gardner Trailhead, the PCT crosses the ridge at a saddle at 9,300 feet just east of Tryon Peak and begins descending toward Noble Lake as you enter the Humboldt-Toiyabe National Forest.

You can see Noble Lake in the distance from the trail, but if you find yourself lakeside you've gone too far. Look for the Bull Canyon Trail on the right that heads to Bull Canyon, where you'll say goodbye to the ease of the PCT's reliable trail condition and count on your own wits to bring you back to the parking lot at the end of the day.

This area is heavily used by cattle, and it's easy to find yourself on a lone cow path that suddenly vanishes. The Bull Canyon Trail climbs up from the PCT to the hike's high point at 9,479 feet, before the dusty, steep descent into Bull Canyon and Wolf Creek. Enjoy the view at the top because it's one of the last vistas on this hike—the remainder of the trail weaves through thick conifer forest and meadow.

My best advice is to stay on the left side of the meadow. However, when I was there, a nursing heifer made this impossible, and I was forced to retreat to the right side. I was still able to connect to the trail by following the riparian vegetation.

As the trail enters deep forest, there is an unmarked fork near mile 6. The trail to the right leads up to Bull Lake, a popular destination for day hikers coming from Wolf Creek but not the most direct way to complete this loop hike. Continue to the left (east) on the Bull Canyon Trail.

The trail braids a thousand times, and in the midst of thick forest it can be hard to keep your head about you. Exactly 0.5 miles past a major stream crossing there is a cabin and a trail leading off to the right; while this shortcut will cut about 2 miles off this loop hike, you'd miss the waterfall on Wolf Creek.

Continue following the braided paths downhill until you reach the Wolf Creek Trail—it feels like a highway after the descent; follow the Wolf Creek Trail right (south). Approximately 0.5 miles from this junction is the fantastic double-drop waterfalls and swimming pools.

The top cascade drops about four feet into a small, deep, and refreshing pool. The second cascade drops about 25 feet into a larger but slightly shallower pool. The top pool is much easier to reach, while reaching the bottom pool requires a little rock climbing. After leaving the falls, the trail enters the meadow within a mile. From here, my best advice is to stay on the trail that parallels Wolf Creek along the creek's west side, but not necessarily within sight of the creek. If you're lucky, around mile 9 you'll come to a trail intersection and signpost that directs traffic left (east) to Murray Canyon and right (west) on the

Elder Creek Trail back uphill to Wolf Creek Pass. Follow the trail to Wolf Creek Pass. Eventually, it intersects the PCT on which you can continue to Highland Lakes.

DIRECTIONS Follow CA 89 south through Markleeville 6 miles to the junction with CA 4; bear right. Follow CA 4 to the top of Ebbetts Pass, 16 miles from the junction. Exactly 1 mile west of Ebbetts Pass there is a road and a sign to Highland Lakes on the left. Follow this road 7 miles to Highland Lakes. After Bloomfield Campground the paved road becomes a dirt road the rest of the way uphill to Highland Lakes Campground. Pass Tryon Meadow Trailhead on the right (west) and turn left into the Gardner Meadow Trailhead parking lot before reaching Highland Lakes.

PERMITS Free wilderness permits are required for overnight trips in Carson-Iceberg Wilderness and can be obtained at the Ebbetts Pass Trailhead as an exception to the in-person permit pick-up policy. The Ebbetts Pass Trailhead is located at the crest of CA 4, east of the road to Highland Lakes. Permits can be obtained at the Calaveras Ranger Station (see page 175 for contact details). Groups are limited to 15 persons and no more than 25 horses or other pack stock.

GPS Trailhead Coordinates	7 Wolf Creek
UTM Zone (WGS 84)	11S
Easting	0256218
Northing	4264646
Latitude	N38° 29.8101′
Longitude	W119° 47.7215′

8 Ebbetts Pass to Upper Kinney Lake

SCENERY: ☆ ☆ ☆ ☆ ☆	DISTANCE: *4.8 miles round-trip*
TRAIL CONDITION: ☆ ☆ ☆ ☆ ☆	HIKING TIME: *2–4 hours*
CHILDREN: ☆ ☆ ☆ ☆ ☆	MAP: *USFS A Guide to the Mokelumne Wilderness*
DIFFICULTY: ☆	
SOLITUDE: ☆ ☆	OUTSTANDING FEATURES: *Upper Kinney Lake, Ebbetts Peak, mountain views*

Hiking to Upper Kinney Lake is a great way to enjoy the afternoon, the sunset, or a night out with the family. This no-fuss, short, and pretty hike teems with wildflowers in midsummer and features breathtaking views into the rugged Eastern Sierra and the Great Basin Range. Upper Kinney's placid waters are an excellent mirror for reflecting the alpenglow off Silver Peak and provide opportunities for fishing (when stocked) and swimming.

👣 Don't be surprised if you hear a cowbell or two from the Ebbetts Pass Trailhead, located on the south side of CA 4 less than a mile east of Ebbetts Pass. Summer cattle grazing is an integral part of the Ebbetts Pass environment and has been for decades. Follow the Ebbetts Pass Trail 0.2 miles until it diverges from the Pacific Crest Trail, where you head right (north). In less than a mile, you cross CA 4 and begin climbing toward the east side of Ebbetts Peak.

Ebbetts Peak is a steep, crumbling granite knob that stands 9,140 feet in elevation. An American flag whips in the wind on its peak and inspires the adventurous to summit the steep feature (a good "first" peak for younger hikers as the off-trail route to the top is only around 400 or so feet of easy, scree scrambling).

The PCT does not cross Ebbetts Peak but rather climbs gradually from its intersection with the highway and passes the small Sherrold and Dorothy lakes. The best way to the peak is from the south side of the lakes directly between the PCT and Ebbetts Peak and then up

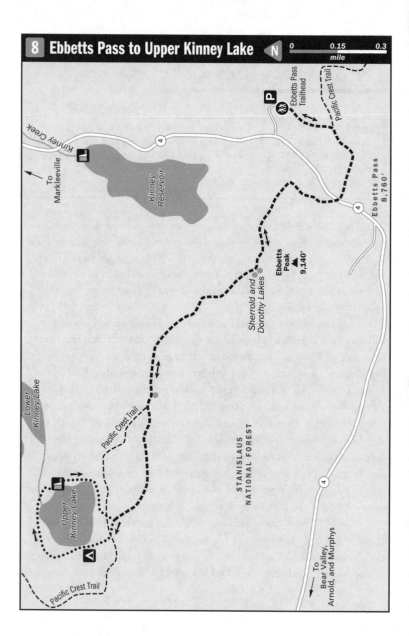

N

0   0.15   0.3
mile

To Markleeville

Kinney Creek

Kinney Reservoir

4

Ebbetts Pass Trailhead

P

Pacific Crest Trail

Ebbetts Pass 8,760'

4

Ebbetts Peak 9,140'

Sherrold and Dorothy Lakes

STANISLAUS NATIONAL FOREST

Lower Kinney Lake

Pacific Crest Trail

Upper Kinney Lake

Pacific Crest Trail

4

To Bear Valley, Arnold, and Murphys

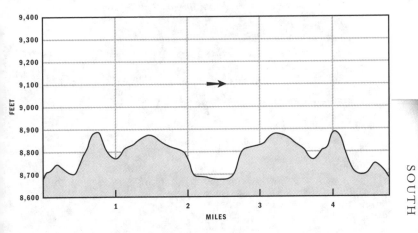

the ridge. The climb is mostly volcanic scree scrambling, and can be done without ropes.

For those more interested in a nice walk, that's exactly what this section of the PCT is—smooth, sandy, hard-packed trail without any loose rock. Bouquets of alpine blossoms—lupines, gooseberry, and mariposa lilies, to name a few—decorate the sides of the trail in midsummer, and views of the jagged ridgelines of Reynolds Peak and Raymond Peak open up to the north. After exactly 2 miles there is a trail intersection for Upper and Lower Kinney lakes. The best camp-sites are straight ahead on the west side of Upper Kinney Lake. This is also a great spot to catch the alpenglow of Silver Peak reflected in the smooth waters of Upper Kinney Lake.

Upper and Lower Kinney Lakes are artificial lakes created by dams constructed in 1926. The Upper Kinney Lake dam holds water from snowmelt in the Silver Creek basin for irrigation purposes downstream on the Carson River and provides water for Lower Kinney Lake 150 feet below. With this said, keep in mind that hikers arriving later in the summer might arrive at Upper Kinney Lake to find it nearly empty.

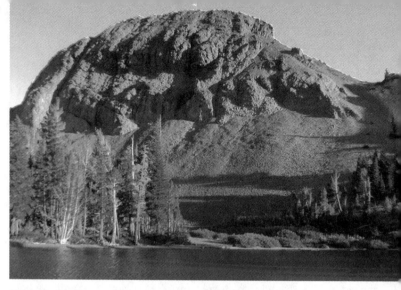

Ebbetts Peak makes a nice detour on the way to Upper Kinney Lake.

DIRECTIONS   Traveling west on CA 4 from Markleeville, the Ebbetts Pass Trailhead is on the left, exactly 5 miles past U.S. Forest Service Silver Creek Campground. Eastbound on CA 4 from Arnold, the trailhead is on the right less than a mile east of Ebbetts Pass.

PERMITS   Backcountry permits are not required for overnight trips to Upper Kinney Lake. Campfire permits are required and can be obtained at any ranger or Cal Fire station. Hikers traveling north of Upper Kinney Lake into the Mokelumne Wilderness need a permit. Self-issued permits are available at the Ebbetts Pass Trailhead. Groups are limited to 8 people for overnight and group size for day use is 12 people.

GPS Trailhead Coordinates	8 Ebbetts Pass to Upper Kinney Lake
UTM Zone (WGS 84)	11S
Easting	0255468
Northing	4270405
Latitude	N38° 32.9085′
Longitude	W119° 48.3580′

9 Carson Pass to Fourth of July Lake

SCENERY: ✰ ✰ ✰ ✰ ✰	HIKING TIME: *7–10 hours or 2 days*
TRAIL CONDITION: ✰ ✰ ✰ ✰ ✰	MAP: *USFS* A Guide to the Mokelumne Wilderness
CHILDREN: ✰ ✰	
DIFFICULTY: ✰ ✰ ✰ ✰	OUTSTANDING FEATURES: *Sweeping mountain vistas, Fourth of July, Winnemucca, and Round Top lakes*
SOLITUDE: ✰ ✰ ✰	
DISTANCE: *14.5 miles round-trip*	

This 14.5-mile loop provides nonstop mountain vistas and features three very pretty alpine lakes, all good for camping, swimming, and fishing. Snow usually flies early on Carson Pass, but if you happen to catch the autumn window between summer and snow, expect to find much of the hike's plant life draped in showy golden hues.

🏃🏃 From the visitor center it's approximately a 1-mile hike on the Pacific Crest Trail to the turnoff to Frog Lake. After another 0.5 miles you'll come to an unmarked fork. A left turn will begin your loop around Elephants Back and Round Top to Fourth of July Lake. For a more direct route to Fourth of July Lake (as well as Winnemucca and Round Top lakes) continue straight on the trail. To complete the circumnavigation loop, bear left to continue south on the PCT.

The PCT drops steeply off the side of Elephants Back over a sunny, treeless hillside. From here the ample views east into the Humboldt-Toiyabe National Forest are incredible as you wind down the trail underneath steep cliffs on the east side of Elephants Back. There's a small creek that irrigates the first valley you'll cross. Expect to see a series of unmarked intersections along the way.

Keep in mind that, excluding the first one, you need to make all right-hand turns to complete this loop. After climbing again past the creek, you come to an intersection with the Summit City Creek Trail.

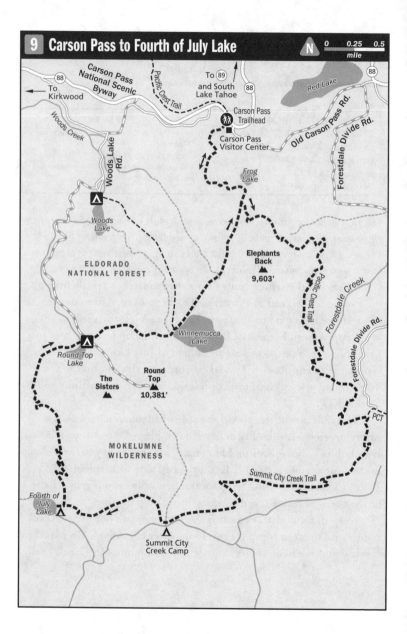

N

0   0.25   0.5
mile

To Kirkwood

Carson Pass National Scenic Byway

88

Woods Creek

Pacific Crest Trail

To 89 and South Lake Tahoe

88

Red Lake

88

Carson Pass Trailhead

Carson Pass Visitor Center

Old Carson Pass Rd.

Woods Lake Rd.

Frog Lake

Forestdale Divide Rd.

Woods Lake

ELDORADO NATIONAL FOREST

Elephants Back
▲
9,603'

Pacific Crest Trail

Forestdale Creek

Winnemucca Lake

Round Top Lake

The Sisters
▲

Round Top
▲
10,381'

Forestdale Divide Rd.

PCT

MOKELUMNE WILDERNESS

Summit City Creek Trail

Fourth of July Lake

Summit City Creek Camp

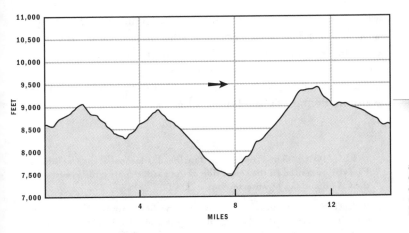

Leave the PCT here and turn right at this four-way intersection toward Summit City Canyon.

The trail swiftly descends the shrubby, balmy south-facing slope while views of the jagged mountains to the south dominate the view. The trail is heavily forested as it parallels Summit City Creek, which was a mining area in the 1800s. Just before an intersection with the trail going right up the back side of Sisters Peak to Fourth of July Lake, there is a nice campsite along the creek. Even better camping awaits at Fourth of July Lake, just a mile's climb above.

Arriving at Fourth of July Lake via Summit City Creek takes 10 miles (as opposed to 5 miles on the front side of Round Top). Regardless of the way you get there, it's a worthy destination for both campers and ambitious day hikers.

Set up camp at one of the handful of established sites around the lake and enjoy the rest of the day and evening fishing or swimming in the lake's deep blue waters. Set at 8,000 feet, this lake is a little chilly but will feel good after a hot summer's day hike.

Expect an early sunset as steep mountain peaks circle the west side of the lake, creating a constant breeze over the waters. Day hikers will want to enjoy the view and location before continuing on the trail up toward Round Top Lake—a 1,200-foot climb in just 2 miles. It's the most difficult leg of the hike, but views of Fourth of July Lake from above take away some of the uphill pain.

For folks looking for a two-day trip, there's also plenty of camping around Round Top and Winnemucca lakes.

DIRECTIONS   The Carson Pass Trailhead is located at the Carson Pass visitor center on the south side of the road, exactly 9 miles west of the CA 88 and CA 89 intersection on CA 88.

PERMITS   Wilderness permits are required year-round for overnight trips in the Carson Pass Management Area and must be obtained in person at the Carson Pass visitor center on CA 88. Camping in the area is available only at Round Top, Winnemucca, and Fourth of July lakes and is *not* permitted at Frog Lake. Permits are given only on a first-come, first-served basis. The visitor center is open daily from 8 a.m. to 4:30 p.m.

GPS Trailhead Coordinates	9 Carson Pass to Fourth of July Lake
UTM Zone (WGS 84)	11S
Easting	0240006
Northing	4287189
Latitude	N38° 41.7081'
Longitude	W119° 59.3665'

10 Carson Pass to Winnemucca Lake

SCENERY: ☆ ☆ ☆ ☆	DISTANCE: *7.7 miles as a loop,*
TRAIL CONDITION: ☆ ☆ ☆ ☆	*4.8 miles with shuttle*
CHILDREN: ☆ ☆ ☆ ☆	HIKING TIME: *2–4 hours*
DIFFICULTY: ☆ ☆	MAP: *USFS* A Guide to the Mokelumne
SOLITUDE: ☆ ☆	Wilderness
	OUTSTANDING FEATURES: *Rugged mountain*
	views, subalpine lakes, especially Winnemucca Lake

This hike can be done as a loop, but parking a shuttle vehicle at Woods Lake Camp-ground shaves about 2 miles off hiking along dirt roads paralleling busy CA 88. Either way, views of dramatic Eldorado National Forest and Mokelumne Wilderness as well as a couple of picturesque lakes will not disappoint.

🏃 Access a short section of the Pacific Crest Trail at the Carson Pass visitor center on the crest of CA 88. This historic summit marks the pass Kit Carson crossed with John C. Frémont during the first government expedition over the Sierra Nevada. More information and a handful of gifts, as well as maps and trail information, are offered inside the visitor center.

Parking fees are $3 per day. If the visitor center is closed, fees can be dropped in an iron ranger at the trailhead. Make a weekend out of it and stay in one of the designated campsites at either Round Top Lake or Winnemucca Lake. Permits are required and must be obtained at the Carson Pass visitor center.

Pick up the trail next to the visitor center and enter a sheltered alpine conifer forest strewn with beautiful granite boulders on either side. The PCT undulates through the forest up a gradual climb before reaching a triangle junction approximately 1 mile from the start.

It's worth it to take the short spur trail left to Frog Lake, a small alpine pond poised on a tabletop with views of Red Lake and CA 88 to the northeast and formidable Round Top to the southwest. The

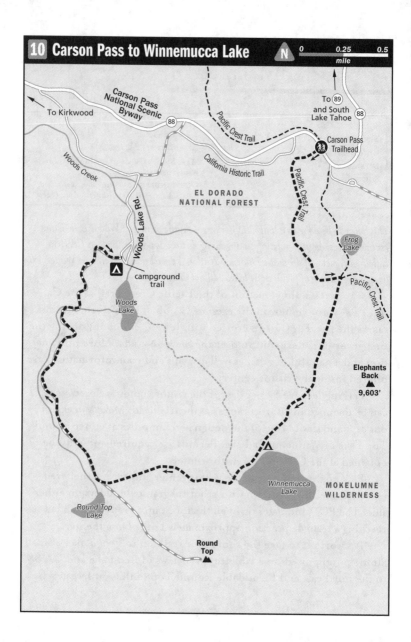

N

0	0.25	0.5

mile

Carson Pass
National Scenic
Byway

To Kirkwood

88

Pacific Crest Trail

To 89
and South
Lake Tahoe

88

Carson Pass
Trailhead

California Historic Trail

Woods Creek

EL DORADO
NATIONAL FOREST

Pacific Crest Trail

Frog
Lake

Woods Lake Rd.

campground
trail

Woods
Lake

Pacific Crest Trail

Elephants
Back
9,603'

Winnemucca
Lake

MOKELUMNE
WILDERNESS

Round Top
Lake

Round
Top

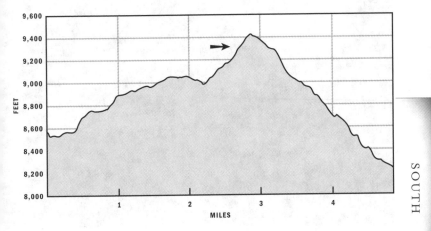

best view of Frog Lake is from its east side. Frog Lake is the midpoint destination for many CA 88 travelers who pull off the highway to stretch their legs.

But for even more spectacular views, after snapping a few photos at Frog Lake continue south to Winnemucca Lake. Follow the trail alongside Frog Lake back to the triangle and go left.

Keep your eyes on Round Top and it's unlikely that you will steer wrong. The trail continues up 0.5 miles or so before coming to another V. Here, the PCT goes to the left, while a well-worn trail to Winnemucca Lake continues right. For this hike, head right. A left turn would take you around a mound dubbed Elephants Back. This trail essentially circumnavigates Round Top by following Summit City Creek on the east side of the mountain and circling around by Fourth of July Lake (see Hike 9, page 59).

For now, take the trail to the right and keep Elephants Back on your left for a nice day-hike option as well as excellent views. You'll soon come to Winnemucca Lake shimmering in the foreground as the rocky and steep Round Top rises right out of its south shore. At

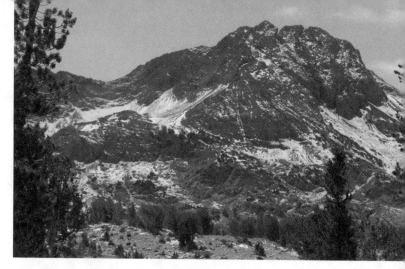

Round Top dominates the landscape on the hike to Winnemucca Lake.

lake level, a maze of a dozen or more spur trails crisscross. Be sure to
stay on a trail because the vegetation in this subalpine environment
is very fragile. Day hikers should continue past the north side of the
lake. Camping is available around the lake with an overnight permit,
which must be obtained from the Carson Pass visitor center at the
trailhead.

On the north side of the lake, you cross a shallow stream and
see a signpost pointing toward Woods Lake. A right turn brings you
directly to Woods Lake via a gradual descent. Follow the trail south,
and after a steady climb from Winnemucca Lake you reach a shallow saddle and a row of high mountains towering above the smaller
Round Top Lake. Camping is also available here. Day hikers turn
right at the signpost pointing toward Woods Lake and follow a steep
creek bed before passing Lost Cabin Mine, an abandoned shaft and
dilapidated structure. Shortly after the historic remnants, the narrow
singletrack merges with an old two-track mining road. Although the

trail never actually passes Woods Lake at lake level, you'll have a view of it from the trail before merging with the road. Once you reach the road, stay right and continue descending.

The trail finally comes to a fork. No matter which way you turn you'll wind up in the Woods Lake Campground parking lot, but the trail to the left is more interesting than the paved campground road. The trail meets the campground road immediately before a small stream crossing and right next to the Woods Lake Campground parking lot. It's best to drop a shuttle vehicle at the campground prior to hiking to avoid returning by foot along the highway.

DIRECTIONS TO TRAILHEAD   Carson Pass is the crest of CA 88. Located 63 miles east of Jackson and approximately 10 miles west of Hope Valley, the Carson Pass visitor center and parking area are on the south side of the highway.

DIRECTIONS FOR SHUTTLE   The Woods Lake Campground is approximately 2 miles west of the Carson Pass visitor center on CA 88 on the south side of the highway. Follow Woods Lake Road to the campground parking lot.

PERMITS   Wilderness permits are required year-round for overnight trips in the Carson Pass Management Area, which must be obtained in person at the Carson Pass visitor center on CA 88. Camping in the area is available only at Round Top and Winnemucca lakes and is not permitted at Frog Lake. Permits are given only on a first-come, first-served basis. The visitor center is open daily from 8 a.m. to 4:30 p.m.

GPS Trailhead Coordinates	10 Carson Pass to Winnemucca Lake
UTM Zone (WGS 84)	10S
Easting	0240409
Northing	4284858
Latitude	N38° 67.4310′
Longitude	W119° 98.3920′

11 Carson Pass to Showers Lake

SCENERY: ☆ ☆ ☆ ☆ ☆	HIKING TIME: *4–6 hours or overnight*
TRAIL CONDITION: ☆ ☆ ☆ ☆ ☆	MAP: Lake Tahoe Basin Trail Map *by*
CHILDREN: ☆ ☆ ☆ ☆	*Adventure Maps*
DIFFICULTY: ☆ ☆ ☆	OUTSTANDING FEATURES: *Incredible*
SOLITUDE: ☆ ☆	*wildflowers, lush mountain meadows, sweeping*
DISTANCE: *10.2 miles round-trip*	*vistas, Showers Lake*

What a great out-and-back hike! This fast, moderately difficult walk wanders through rustling aspen groves, bucolic meadows, and along mountain ridges providing stunning views of this lush high country. Take this hike in mid-July to mid-August to enjoy a vibrant display of beautiful wildflowers.

🏃🏃 Make sure to bring either cash or check to the trailhead to pay the $5-per-day parking fee. You won't miss the drop box; it's located right at the trailhead. This hike follows the Pacific Crest Trail.

For the first 0.5 miles, the trail meanders through a few rustling aspen groves and stands of pine. For the next mile, the well-traveled, sandy trail climbs gradually up the treeless slope on the side of Red Lake Peak through fields of sage and mule's ears. As you crest the rise you'll get a glimpse of Lake Tahoe before descending into the headwaters of the Upper Truckee River and Meiss Meadows.

After 3.5 miles, the PCT intersects the Tahoe Rim Trail, which leads to Round Lake, 2 miles away. At this point, Showers Lake is also 2 miles away straight ahead on the PCT. At this intersection is also the still-standing homestead of Louis Meiss, who immigrated to California from Germany in the mid-1800s. The barn and house, which were the summer grazing grounds for Meiss's cattle, were built in 1878 and abandoned in the 1930s. Seeing a home in such an amazing place gives a fantastic perspective. While cattle no longer graze these meadows, the cowboy legacy is still intact. This trail is popular with backcountry equestrians.

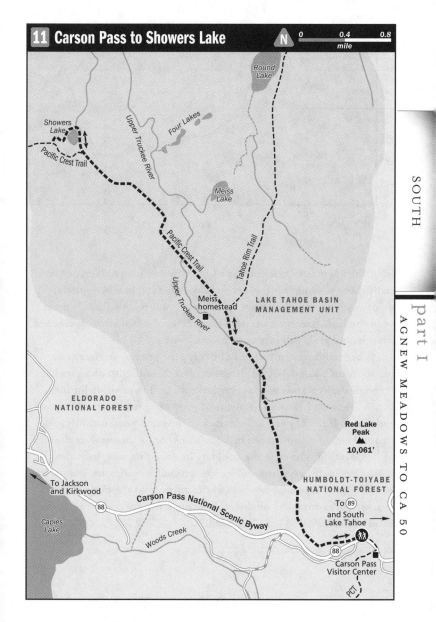

Round
Lake

Showers
Lake

Upper Truckee River

Four Lakes

Pacific Crest Trail

Meiss
Lake

Pacific Crest Trail

Tahoe Rim Trail

Upper Truckee River

Meiss
homestead

LAKE TAHOE BASIN
MANAGEMENT UNIT

ELDORADO
NATIONAL FOREST

Red Lake
Peak
▲
10,061'

To Jackson
and Kirkwood

Caples
Lake

88

Carson Pass National Scenic Byway

Woods Creek

HUMBOLDT-TOIYABE
NATIONAL FOREST

To 89
and South
Lake Tahoe →

88

Carson Pass
Visitor Center

PCT

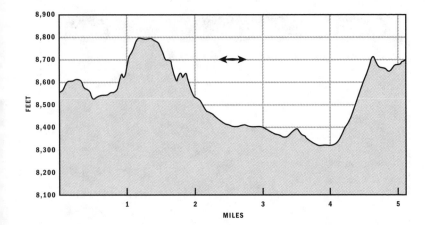

Meiss Meadows is the destination point for many hikers, especially those seeking wildflowers. It looks like God had fun splattering paint as white, yellow, orange, pink, blue, and purple flowers meld onto the lush, green canvas of the meadow. Watching the breeze race over the tall grass will take your breath away.

The trail ducks in and out of shady pine groves—perfect resting spots on a hot day—and climbs the last 0.5 miles to Showers Lake through showy stands of towering larkspur and royal-blue lupines.

At Showers Lake there's plenty of good camping if you can't force yourself to leave. It's easy to lose track of time and responsibility at this pastoral scene. A lush, green meadow slopes onto Showers' south side, while gleaming, white granite boulders line the west side, providing private nooks for camping and a nice bottom for testing the waters.

The cool water in Showers Lake is murky and the bottom is mucky, but around the boulders there are a few good spots to go for a swim without getting your feet muddy.

DIRECTIONS   From South Lake Tahoe, take CA 89 south to the intersection of CA 88. Turn right and head west 9.5 miles to the trailhead on
the right, just after Carson Pass and the Carson Pass visitor center. Traveling east on CA 88, you reach the trailhead on the left 5.4 miles after the
turn to Kirkwood Mountain Resort.

PERMITS   Backcountry permits are not required for overnight trips to
Showers Lake. Campfire permits are required and can be obtained at any
ranger or Cal Fire station.

GPS Trailhead Coordinates	11 Carson Pass to Showers Lake
UTM Zone (WGS 84)	11S
Easting	0239800
Northing	4287379
Latitude	N38° 41.8074′
Longitude	W119° 59.5128′

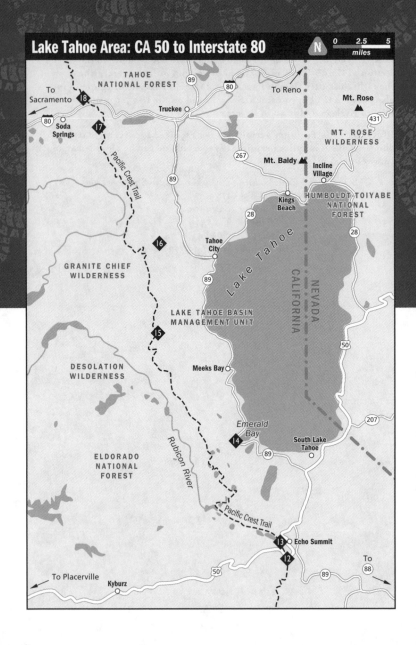

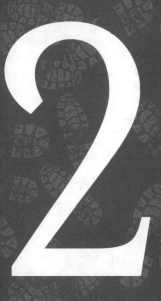

2

LAKE TAHOE AREA

12 Echo Summit to Meiss Meadows Overlook

SCENERY: ✿ ✿ ✿	DISTANCE: *4.3 miles round-trip*
TRAIL CONDITION: ✿ ✿ ✿ ✿	HIKING TIME: *2 hours*
CHILDREN: ✿ ✿ ✿ ✿	MAP: Lake Tahoe Basin Trail Map *by Adventure Maps*
DIFFICULTY: ✿	
SOLITUDE: ✿ *(depending on season)*	OUTSTANDING FEATURES: *Wildlife, fall colors, alpine meadows*

This short trip gets the heart pumping with a nice climb to a beautiful overlook, but for an extremely mellow, short hike go no farther than Benwood Meadow.

The trail starts at the west end of the Pacific Crest Trailhead parking lot at the top of Echo Summit. Most foot traffic takes a right at the trailhead and crosses US 50 toward stunning Echo Lakes. Heading left at the trailhead instead takes you toward beautiful mountain meadows. Both hikes are outstanding, but for slightly less traffic and a shorter hike, head left toward the meadows.

Approximately 100 yards from the start, make a hairpin right turn to continue on the PCT and Tahoe Rim Trail. The trail parallels the Echo Summit Cross Country Ski Center parking lot and weaves in and out of cross-country ski trails. The trail turns into a doublewide track for a short while before a small singletrack trail marked with the PCT emblem veers off to the right. Go right. The trail ascends through a rocky Christmas-tree forest popular with mountain bikers, so beware.

The trail intersects with another doubletrack and continues uphill before making a left onto a small singletrack trail marked with the PCT emblem. It might seem confusing, but it's actually pretty intuitive when you're there. The trail continues to ramble (though

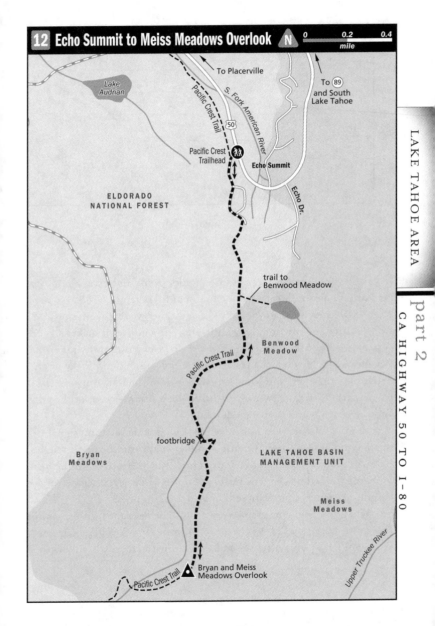

N

0   0.2   0.4
mile

To Placerville

S. Fork American River

To 89
and South
Lake Tahoe

Lake
Audrian

Pacific Crest Trail

50

Pacific Crest
Trailhead

Echo Summit

Echo Dr.

ELDORADO
NATIONAL FOREST

trail to
Benwood Meadow

Benwood
Meadow

Pacific Crest Trail

footbridge

Bryan
Meadows

LAKE TAHOE BASIN
MANAGEMENT UNIT

Meiss
Meadows

Upper Truckee River

Pacific Crest Trail

Bryan and Meiss
Meadows Overlook

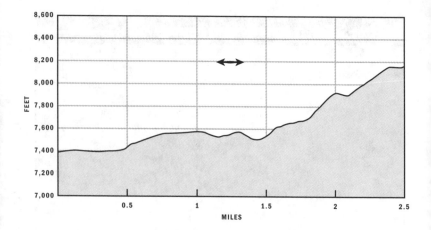

less aimlessly) through large granite boulders and tight trees before reaching Benwood Meadow after 1 mile of hiking.

A little spur trail connects to the meadows, visible from the PCT. A nice spot to sit quietly and watch for wildlife, it makes a good destination for hikers interested in a short, easy, and pretty hike. Past Benwood Meadow the trail hugs the bottom end of blocky, granite cliffs to the right and low-lying meadows to the left. Autumn is a particularly nice time to take this hike, when summer crowds dwindle and the aspen leaves turn a golden hue.

At mile 1.4 a newer footbridge crosses a seasonal stream, signaling the impending climb. Granite boulder stairs lead the way up to the Bryan and Meiss meadows overlook at just over 8,000 feet. In the next mile, the trail climbs approximately 800 feet while eagles screech and chipmunks scurry in this incredibly wild-looking area.

When the trail comes to its crest you'll be rewarded with splendid views into Bryan and Meiss meadows, but the views are better up on the left. Pick a point off-trail and walk along the sturdy boulders to find the crest of the hillside for a breathtaking perch over the meadows. From here, turn around and go back the way you came in. For a longer trip, Bryan Meadows is approximately 2 miles ahead.

DIRECTIONS From Meyers (near South Lake Tahoe), look for the left turnoff to the Pacific Crest Trailhead just after cresting Echo Summit.

GPS Trailhead Coordinates	12 Echo Summit to Meiss Meadows Overlook
UTM Zone (WGS 84)	10S
Easting	0757525
Northing	4300370
Latitude	N38° 48.8690′
Longitude	W120° 02.0400′

13 Echo Lake to Lake Aloha

SCENERY: ✪ ✪ ✪ ✪ ✪
TRAIL CONDITION: ✪ ✪ ✪ ✪
CHILDREN: ✪ ✪ ✪ ✪ ✪
DIFFICULTY: ✪ ✪
SOLITUDE: ✪
DISTANCE: 6 miles round-trip with boat shuttle both ways; 12 miles round-trip without

HIKING TIME: 2–5 hours
MAP: Lake Tahoe Basin Trail Map by Adventure Maps
OUTSTANDING FEATURES: Lake Aloha, wildflowers, boat shuttle, cozy cottages tucked into the lakeshore

What a charming day hike! You'll forget the splendor of Tahoe once you've hiked from camp-y Echo Lakes to face-of-the-moon Lake Aloha. One of the highlights is taking the boat shuttle, at least one way, from the parking lot at Lower Echo Lake. This is a great hike for families.

🚶🚶 Echo Lake's idyllic setting is the summer home for a handful of fortunate folks whose forefathers happened to be at the right place at the right time. During the 1930s, the U.S. Forest Service released a limited number of lease properties on the lake. At this time (or as the story goes), a handful of professors from the University of California, Berkeley happened to be in the area and heard news of the leases up for grabs. Word traveled quickly to friends in Berkeley and what has resulted is an Echo Lakes community or club, if you will, that is made up primarily of Berkeley folks.

While enjoying Echo Lake is completely open to the public, if you want to spend a weekend in one of the enchanting lakeside cottages you'll have to "know somebody." Lease restrictions do not allow homeowners to rent out their cottages. However, Echo Lake Chalets (www.echochalet.com) *does* rent cottages just off the lake during the summer.

The novelty of this hike is that the trail can be accessed by boat shuttle, which I highly recommend. The shuttle leaves "when full," which on nice summer days is generally no longer than 30 minutes between shuttles. Operating hours are Memorial Day through Labor

Tallac Creek

Dicks Lake

LAKE TAHOE BASIN MANAGEMENT UNIT

▲ **Mt. Tallac**

Fallen Leaf Lake

Cathedral Creek

Half Moon Lake

Pacific Crest Trail

Gilmore Lake

Glen Alpine Trail

Glen Alpine Creek

DESOLATION WILDERNESS

Susie Lake

Fallen Leaf Rd.

Angora Ridge Rd.

Heather Lake

Lake Aloha

Cracked Crag

Glen Alpine Creek

Angora Creek

N. Upper Truckee Rd.

Lake Margery

Lake Lucille

▲ **Angora Peak**

Angora Lakes

Keiths Dome ▲

trail to Triangle Lake

▲ **Echo Peak**

▲ **Pyramid Peak**

Lake of the Woods

Tahoe Rim Trail/PCT

To South Lake Tahoe

Tamarack Lake

boat taxi dock

Upper Echo Lake

Lower Echo Lake

50

Ralston Peak ▲

▲ **Talking Mtn.**

🚶 ⚓

P   Echo Lakes Rd.

Becker Peak ▲

Pyramid Creek

DESOLATION WILDERNESS

50

Tamarack Creek

Aspen Creek

Pacific Crest Trail

50

Bryant Creek

ELDORADO NATIONAL FOREST

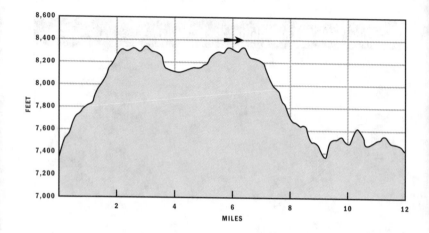

Day, daily from 8 a.m. to 6:30 p.m. Taxi rides are $10 per person each way; dogs ride for $5. From the marina at the Echo Lake parking lot tickets can be purchased with cash or a credit card. From the drop-off at the end of Upper Echo Lake, there is a drop phone to call for a taxi during operating hours. If the drop phone doesn't work, there is also a credit-card-only pay phone. Maximum wait time for a taxi at the far end is generally no longer than 30 minutes as well.

The boat taxi turns approximately one hour of rolling hiking on the PCT along Echo Lake into about 15 minutes. My recommendation is to take the boat taxi at least one way, probably on the way back when you've had your fill of hiking.

To pick up the PCT from the Echo Lakes marina parking lot, cross the dam to reach the trailhead. This section of the PCT is also the Tahoe Rim Trail; follow the trail northwest hugging Lower and Upper Echo Lakes.

Or, if you choose to start from the dock at the end of Upper Echo Lake, follow the trail up the hill past the pay phone and make a left on the combination PCT/TRT.

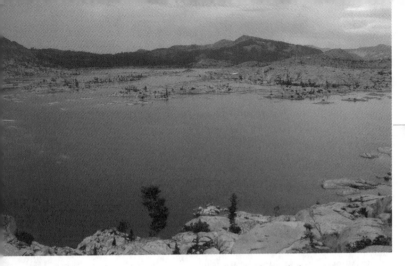

Lake Aloha, set at 8,200 feet, is dotted with hundreds of smooth, barren, granite islands.

The trail climbs steadily over loose rock past Tamarack Lake below until the second turnoff to Triangle Lake, where it flattens out into a nice hard-packed path through wildflowers (midsummer), meadow, and forest. Along the way there are options to make side trips to Triangle Lake, Tamarack Lake, Lake of the Woods, and Lake Lucille. Shortly after passing Lake Margery, which you can see from the trail, the trail begins descending to Lake Aloha. Less than a mile from Lake Aloha the trail splits, each way pointing to Lake Aloha. The right is a slightly more direct approach; going left is slightly better swimming and more private.

Lake Aloha is a massive, shallow lake dotted with hundreds of smooth, barren, granite islands. Once known as Medley Lakes, Lake Aloha is a reservoir that supplies water to the Eldorado irrigation system. To thoroughly make the most of your day hike to Lake Aloha (which could easily be extended to an overnight if you can't bear to leave), pack an inflatable raft and paddle. Paddling around is an excellent way to explore the vastness of this backcountry lake with all of its inlets, secret beaches, and interesting islands. From your first sighting of the lake, it's impossible to see its scope. Hiking along the PCT for about another mile alongside the lake provides a clearer picture. Spend the day swimming, lay on the ubiquitous granite boulders along the lake, or stash your gear and set out on the water to find your own private piece of paradise.

DIRECTIONS   Following US 50 west of South Lake Tahoe, turn right on Johnson Pass Road exactly 1 mile after Echo Summit. You will see a brown sign pointing to Echo Lake. Follow Johnson Pass Road 0.5 miles before turning left onto Echo Lakes Road. There is also a sign pointing to Atwood Tract at this intersection.

Follow Echo Lakes Road 1.3 miles to the parking lot at Echo Lake. On busy summer days, the lot might be full. If so, simply park on the side of the road.

PERMITS   Day and overnight use permits are required for travel in the Desolation Wilderness. Hikers can issue themselves a day use permit at the trailhead. Overnight permits must be picked up in person at one of the following offices: Lake Tahoe Visitor Center, 3 miles north of the junction of Highways 50 and 89 at South Lake Tahoe on Highway 89, open in summer only, call (530) 543-2674; Lake Tahoe Basin Management Unit, at 35 College Drive in South Lake Tahoe, call (530) 543-2600.

GPS Trailhead Coordinates	13 Echo Lake to Lake Aloha
UTM Zone (WGS 84)	10S
Easting	0756570
Northing	4302580
Latitude	N38° 50.0792'
Longitude	W120° 02.6498'

14 Emerald Bay to Lake Aloha

SCENERY: ✿ ✿ ✿ ✿ ✿	HIKING TIME: *2–3 days*
TRAIL CONDITION: ✿ ✿ ✿ ✿ ✿	MAP: Lake Tahoe Basin Trail Map *by*
CHILDREN: ✿ ✿ ✿	*Adventure Maps*
DIFFICULTY: ✿ ✿ ✿ ✿	OUTSTANDING FEATURES: *Numerous alpine*
SOLITUDE: ✿ ✿	*lakes for swimming, Lake Aloha, outstanding wildflow-*
DISTANCE: *21 miles round-trip*	*ers in the Rubicon drainage, rugged mountain views*

*There's a maze of remarkable trails west of South Lake Tahoe in the rugged Desola-
tion Wilderness. This loop makes a great two-nighter, with plenty of scenic lakes plus
brilliant displays of wildflowers in midsummer, along the way.*

🚶🚶 Before you begin, keep in mind that permits are required
for both day and overnight use in the Desolation Wilderness, see
page 87 for details. This area is one of the most scenic and enjoyable sections of the Pacific Crest Trail in northern California due to
its sheer number of lakes and wildflowers in the summer. This long
loop lets you see the best of it. For a shorter (12-mile) loop, circle
Upper Velma, Fontanillis, and Dicks lakes.

To park at the Eagle Falls Trailhead, you need to pay a $5 over-
night fee at the drop box at the lot. The short (0.75-mile) hike to
Eagle Falls is very popular, so arrive early or late, as opposed to mid-
day, when tourist traffic swells.

The trail climbs steeply from the start for 2 miles past Eagle Falls
and above Eagle Lake before leveling out on the crest. Take your mind
off the exertion by enjoying the stunning views of sunken Eagle Lake.

Shortly after the crest, you'll reach a fork in the trail and your
first glimpses into the vastness of Desolation Wilderness. The trails
are all incredibly well signed, so it's unlikely you'll get lost. For this
loop, head straight to one of my favorite spots, Dicks Lake. For
that route, head right to Velma Lakes at the intersection with the

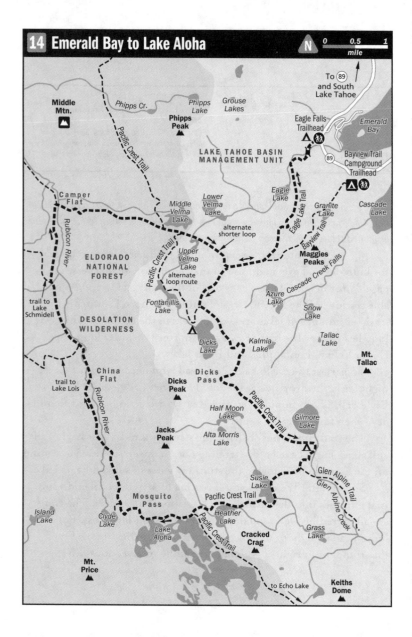

N

0   0.5   1
mile

To (89)
and South
Lake Tahoe

Middle
Mtn.

Phipps Cr.

*Phipps
Lake*

*Grouse
Lakes*

**Phipps
Peak**

Eagle Falls
Trailhead

*Emerald
Bay*

LAKE TAHOE BASIN
MANAGEMENT UNIT

Bayview Trail
Campground
Trailhead

(89)

Pacific Crest Trail

Camper
Flat

*Middle
Velma
Lake*

*Lower
Velma
Lake*

*Eagle
Lake*

*Granite
Lake*

*Cascade
Lake*

Rubicon River

ELDORADO
NATIONAL
FOREST

Pacific Crest Trail

*Upper
Velma
Lake*

alternate
shorter loop

Eagle Lake Trail

Bayview Trail

**Maggies
Peaks**

trail to
Lake Schmidell

DESOLATION
WILDERNESS

alternate
loop route

*Fontanillis
Lake*

Cascade Creek Falls

*Azure
Lake*

*Snow
Lake*

*Dicks
Lake*

*Kalmia
Lake*

*Tallac
Lake*

**Mt.
Tallac**

trail to
Lake Lois

China
Flat

**Dicks
Peak**

Dicks
Pass

Pacific Crest Trail

Rubicon River

*Half Moon
Lake*

*Gilmore
Lake*

**Jacks
Peak**

*Alta Morris
Lake*

Glen Alpine Trail

*Island
Lake*

Mosquito
Pass

Pacific Crest Trail

*Susie
Lake*

Glen Alpine Creek

**Clyde
Lake**

*Lake
Aloha*

Pacific Crest Trail

*Heather
Lake*

**Cracked
Crag**

*Grass
Lake*

**Mt.
Price**

to Echo Lake

**Keiths
Dome**

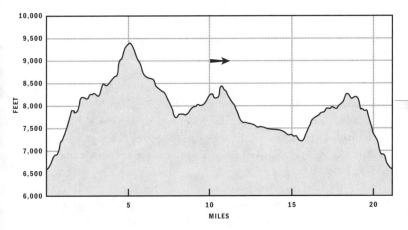

Bayview Trail (a good alternate starting point, see map for details). At the next sign, the trail splits again. A right bearing would take you to Velma Lakes and Rockbound Valley. Bear left toward Dicks Lake.

Dicks Lake, about 4 miles from the start, is a great swimming spot and popular for camping as well. There are plenty of sites around it, but my favorites are on the near side to watch the moon rise over the lake.

After spending a few moments (or the night) at Dicks Lake, continue back to the Pacific Crest Trail up and over Dicks Pass. The wildflowers on the pass are absolutely incredible midsummer. Over the pass and about 8 miles from the start, good camping can be found at Gilmore Lake (especially if you like to fish) and at Half Moon Lake (which is incredibly scenic) if you have only one night to spend in the backcountry.

Shortly after Gilmore Lake, the PCT meets a junction with the Glen Alpine Trail, a popular access point from Fallen Leaf Lake. The PCT travels along Susie and Heather lakes (both better for fishing than swimming), before reaching the breathtaking Lake Aloha.

Lake Aloha is an expansive, shallow alpine lake/reservoir sur-rounded by gray granite beaches as far as the eye can see. It looks like the face of the moon.

After spending the day (or night) at Lake Aloha, continue up the short and mellow Mosquito Pass to complete this loop. You will promptly descend into the headwaters of the Rubicon River and will pass Clyde Lake. Many people decide to take their swim at Clyde Lake instead of Aloha and, I have to say, the idea is tempting. Much smaller and deeper, Clyde Lake is also slightly more scenic than Aloha.

The trail follows the Rubicon drainage for about 7 miles, cross-ing over the creek a few times along the way and gradually descend-ing into Rockbound Valley. In midsummer, this is a jungle of wildflowers. I've never seen such beautiful flowers in my life, but you'll be competing for photo ops with the incessant mosquito population in this low-lying drainage. Bring the bug net, spray, and thick skin! Many people avoid the drainage altogether and simply hike out-and-back to the lakes of their choice, but a loop hike lets you see much more.

Follow the drainage until a sign to Velma Lakes directs you across the creek and back to where you started. A wrong turn here would be to follow the trail into Rockbound Valley.

DIRECTIONS The Eagle Falls Trailhead is 18.6 miles south of Tahoe City (at the Y), on the west (right) side of CA 89. Coming from South Lake Tahoe (at the Y), the trailhead is 8.6 miles north, on the left-hand side of CA 89.

DIRECTIONS TO ALTERNATE TRAILHEAD Many hikers enter this part of Desolation Wilderness via the Bayview Trail. To access, continue up the steep hill on CA 89 south of Emerald Bay and within 1 mile turn into the Bayview Campground on the right-hand side of the

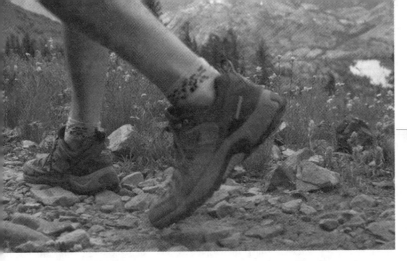

Susie Lake shimmers below while a hiker puts one foot in front of the other on the PCT on Dicks Pass.

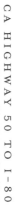
highway. There is a dirt parking lot past the campground at the trailhead. The Bayview Trail is incredibly scenic, with views of pretty Granite Lake and multiple views of Lake Tahoe.

PERMITS   Day and overnight use permits are required for travel in the Desolation Wilderness. Hikers can issue themselves a day use permit at the trailhead. Overnight permits must be picked up in person at one of the following offices: Lake Tahoe Visitor Center, 3 miles north of the junction of Highways 50 and 89 at South Lake Tahoe on Highway 89, open in summer only, call (530) 543-2674; Lake Tahoe Basin Management Unit, at 35 College Drive in South Lake Tahoe, call (530) 543-2600.

GPS Trailhead Coordinates	14 Emerald Bay to Lake Aloha
UTM Zone (WGS 84)	10S
Easting	0750238
Northing	4315462
Latitude	N38° 57.1448′
Longitude	W120° 06.7401′

15 Barker Pass to Twin Peaks

SCENERY: ✿ ✿ ✿ ✿ ✿	DISTANCE: *10.5 miles round-trip*
TRAIL CONDITION: ✿ ✿ ✿ ✿ ✿	HIKING TIME: *4–6 hours*
CHILDREN: ✿ ✿ ✿	MAP: Lake Tahoe Basin Trail Map *by*
DIFFICULTY: ✿ ✿ ✿	*Adventure Maps*
SOLITUDE: ✿ ✿ ✿	OUTSTANDING FEATURES: *Breathtaking views*
DOGS: ✿ ✿ ✿ ✿ ✿	*of Lake Tahoe, giant fir forests, optional*
	peak scramble

Incredible scenery and gentle, varied terrain make this out-and-back journey a half-day delight. The hike follows the well-worn Pacific Crest Trail most of the way. A short side trip on the Tahoe Rim Trail to Twin Peaks is a bonus for the adventurous peak bagger, and a brief talus scramble to the top provides an unforgettable bird's-eye view of Lake Tahoe.

🏃 Although well trod in the summer months, this hike receives far less traffic in the fall when it is arguably at its prettiest. Golden aspen line the road to the trailhead and splash color into Blackwood Canyon.

The trail, which is both the Tahoe Rim Trail and the PCT, begins a gradual climb almost immediately from the Barker Pass Trailhead dirt parking lot, with expansive views into Granite Chief Wilderness. Views into Desolation Wilderness open up to the south as you climb the ridgeline skirting the summit of Barker Pass.

Lake Tahoe views start after exactly 1 mile, where an overlook on the right provides a sweeping vista of Blackwood Ridge and Canyon in the foreground and the giant blue Tahoe in the distance. After this vista, you'll enjoy continuous views of Lake Tahoe. At mile 1.4, a spur trail leads to a volcanic outcrop and excellent lake overlook and photo opportunity. The elevation rises and falls as the trail easily undulates through conifer forests west of Blackwood Canyon, crossing small streams twice.

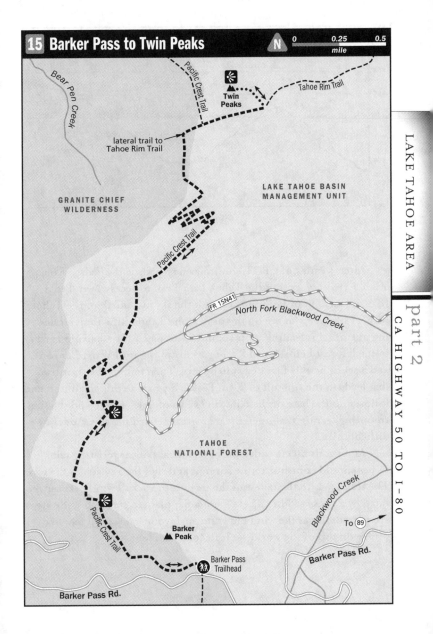

Bear Pen Creek

Pacific Crest Trail

Twin Peaks

Tahoe Rim Trail

lateral trail to
Tahoe Rim Trail

GRANITE CHIEF
WILDERNESS

LAKE TAHOE BASIN
MANAGEMENT UNIT

Pacific Crest Trail

FR 15N4

North Fork Blackwood Creek

TAHOE
NATIONAL FOREST

Blackwood Creek

To 89

Pacific Crest Trail

Barker
Peak

Barker Pass
Trailhead

Barker Pass Rd.

Barker Pass Rd.

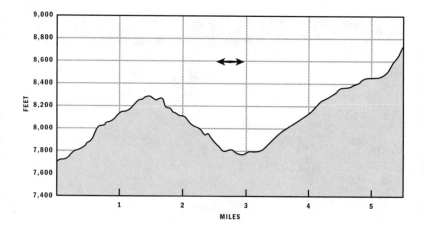

After 4 miles, the PCT continues north while the Tahoe Rim
Trail turns east. Follow the Tahoe Rim Trail to access Twin Peaks
(8,878 feet). Twin Peaks juts up into the sky just north of the Tahoe
Rim Trail. Keep an eye on the peak as the Tahoe Rim Trail circles
the pile of talus leading to its summit, and watch for a hairpin turn
to the left just before the TRT begins dropping into Ward Canyon
and a set of heavily forested switchbacks. Turn left on the spur trail
that leads to the summit of Twin Peaks. If you take this small trail and
follow it to the base of the talus, the views of Lake Tahoe and the surrounding terrain that open up are a great reward for this moderately
difficult hike.

Ambitious hikers with a bit of technical skill negotiating talus
slopes should continue to the summit and sign the registry at the top.
The trail leads to the tallest of the two steep, rocky Twin Peaks sepa-
rated by a rocky saddle. There's not a flat place to stand, but the views
are incredible; as the wind blows through your hair you'll feel like
you're on top of the world—at least for a moment.

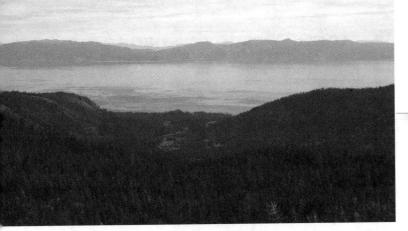

Continuous views of Lake Tahoe make every step of this hike to Twin Peaks enjoyable.

DIRECTIONS From CA 89, turn right on Barker Pass Road (labeled Blackwood Canyon Road on the recommended map) 4.25 miles south of Tahoe City. Follow the road, veering left, 7.2 miles to the dirt parking lot for the PCT and Tahoe Rim Trail.

GPS Trailhead Coordinates	15 Barker Pass to Twin Peaks
UTM Zone (WGS 84)	10S
Easting	0739177
Northing	4328977
Latitude	N39° 04.629'
Longitude	W120° 14.1060'

16 Alpine Meadows Road to Squaw Valley

SCENERY: ✿ ✿ ✿	DISTANCE: *8.25 miles point-to-point*
TRAIL CONDITION: ✿ ✿ ✿ ✿ ✿	HIKING TIME: *4 hours*
CHILDREN: ✿ ✿ ✿ ✿	MAP: Lake Tahoe Basin Trail Map *by*
DIFFICULTY: ✿ ✿	*Adventure Maps*
SOLITUDE: ✿	OUTSTANDING FEATURES: *Five Lakes, Squaw Valley*

This popular point-to-point hike passes a collection of five pretty lakes, aptly named Five Lakes, as it climbs steadily to the back side of Squaw Valley Ski Area. In season, reward yourself with a ride on Squaw Valley's Cable Car to take advantage of superb après-hike food and entertainment in the Village at Squaw.

🚶 Expect to start climbing immediately from the Five Lakes Trailhead. The often-dusty trail cuts back and forth for the first mile across the sunny, shrubby hillside. Just after the first mile, the trail levels off and provides a nice spot for photos or a water break before continuing to Five Lakes or Squaw Valley.

Near the top of this first climb you pass a few chairlift towers on the hillside that are the possession of Sue and Troy Caldwell and part of a work in progress for the Caldwell family private ski area. The trail to Five Lakes passes through the Caldwell's property from the trailhead until the Tahoe National Forest sign. Because of an easement with the U.S. Forest Service, hikers are allowed to travel on the trail as long as they don't stray more than 10 feet in either direction of the trail. After Pritzker Ridge, the trail travels through an area the Caldwells affectionately call "White Wolf" (for a white dog they rescued in the area) for about a half mile to the boundary of the Granite Chief Wilderness and Tahoe National Forest.

Respect the Caldwells' property and stay on the trail through this section. At the end of the property line the trail enters a towering

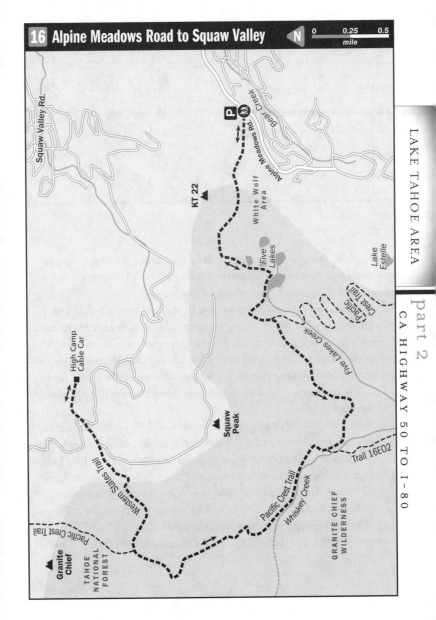

N

0   0.25   0.5
mile

Squaw Valley Rd.

Bear Creek

P 🚶🚶

Alpine Meadows Rd.

KT 22 ▲

White Wolf Area

Five Lakes

Lake Estelle ▲

Pacific Crest Trail

Five Lakes Creek

High Camp Cable Car ■

Squaw Peak ▲

Trail 16E02

Western States Trail

Pacific Crest Trail

Whiskey Creek

GRANITE CHIEF WILDERNESS

Pacific Crest Trail

Granite Chief ▲

TAHOE NATIONAL FOREST

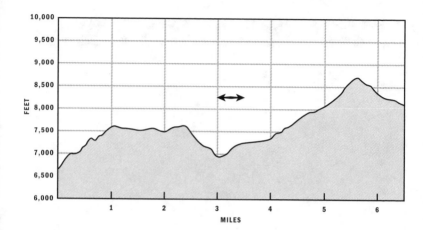

pine forest. Shortly after entering the forest and 1.8 miles from the trailhead you come to an unmarked triangle of trails; turn left (south) at this fork to access the collection of five lakes.

The first and second lakes are small, shallow, and marshy, with vibrant stands of fireweed lining the shoreline in early to midsummer. After the second lake, veer right (west) at the next unmarked fork to access the biggest of the Five Lakes. This lake is suitable for fishing and swimming, and there are also a few flat spots to pitch a tent. Be forewarned that this trail, and especially this lake, is a very popular destination for day hikers.

The trail, which disappears here and there along the lake, mostly follows the shoreline north to the end of the lake, where it resembles a trail again. About 500 yards or so past the biggest of the Five Lakes is another intersection, with a sign pointing left to the Pacific Crest Trail. Follow this trail a short distance to join the PCT 2.7 miles from the trailhead. Take a right and head northwest on the PCT.

The trail crosses a shallow, marshy creek shortly after the intersection with the Five Lakes Trail and descends briefly through a mixed conifer forest and fields of wildflowers—hundreds of bright yellow mountain mule's ears in early to midsummer.

Hikers can access Whiskey Creek Camp and Diamond Crossing on trail 16E02, which intersects the PCT about 3.5 miles south of Granite Chief. To access Squaw, follow the PCT as it climbs toward Granite Chief, offering spectacular views into Whiskey Creek Canyon and beyond. Leave the views to climb through a forest of predominant mountain hemlocks covered in moss from the snow-line up.

After 6 miles of hiking from the Five Lakes Trailhead, you'll see a fork where the Tevis Trail, or the Western States Trail, heads left (west). This trail hosts a popular 100-mile endurance race, which starts at Squaw Valley and finishes in Auburn. Runners tackle this enduro-descent in June, while the horseback riding event is gener-ally held in late July or early August. Continue on the PCT heading north.

In another mile, you break off from the PCT and turn right toward Squaw Valley at a four-way intersection. From here you can clearly see the boundary fence on the ridge above Squaw Valley. Although a few unmarked trails come in here and there, continue right, following the trail on the west side of the ridge up the final climb to the top.

You find a monument celebrating the Placer County Emigrant Road (known today as the Western States Trail), built in 1854 as a connection between the California foothills and the Comstock Lode boom towns of Gold Hill, Silver City, and Virginia City in Nevada's Washoe Valley. The monument stands at the original trail marker constructed by Robert Watson in summer 1931.

From here, a fantastic view of Lake Tahoe stretches before you on the eastern horizon, and numerous chairlifts and service roads crisscross the landscape below. The building farthest left is the Squaw Valley Cable Car building. Follow the dirt roads to High Camp via

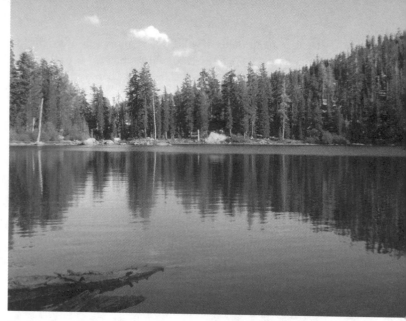

The biggest of the Five Lakes is a great way to cool off in the heat of the day on this popular hike.

Bailey's Beach Camp and hitch a ride on the cable car into the village to celebrate your hike (tickets are $10 per adult).

The cable car is open late June through the end of August from 9:40 a.m. until 9 p.m. Through mid-September, the last car leaves High Camp at 4 p.m. From September 15 through the beginning of winter the cable car is closed. Once Squaw Valley opens for the ski season, the cable car operates from 9 a.m. until 8:40 p.m. on weekends and until 7 p.m. Monday through Thursday. For more information, visit www.squaw.com.

DIRECTIONS From Interstate 80, exit CA 89 south toward Lake Tahoe. In 9.7 miles, turn right on Alpine Meadows Road. Follow the road for 2 miles and look for a wide dirt shoulder on the right-hand side. This is the parking area for the Five Lakes Trailhead.

To set up a shuttle vehicle at Squaw Valley, follow CA 89 8.3 miles south of I-80 and turn right onto Squaw Valley Road at the traffic light. Follow Squaw Valley Road to the village parking area on the left at the end of the road.

GPS Trailhead Coordinates	16 Alpine Meadows Road to Squaw Valley
UTM Zone (WGS 84)	10S
Easting	0739277
Northing	4340310
Latitude	N39° 10.8545′
Longitude	W120° 13.8587′

17 Sugar Bowl to Squaw Valley

SCENERY: ✿ ✿ ✿ ✿	DISTANCE: *11.9 miles point-to-point*
TRAIL CONDITION: ✿ ✿ ✿ ✿	HIKING TIME: *4–6 hours*
CHILDREN: ✿ ✿	MAP: Lake Tahoe Basin Trail Map *by*
DIFFICULTY: ✿ ✿ ✿ ✿	*Adventure Maps*
SOLITUDE: ✿ ✿ ✿	OUTSTANDING FEATURES: *Partial Lake Tahoe views, Squaw Valley*

Linking two of the Tahoe area's popular ski resorts, this 12-mile one-way journey almost exclusively on the Pacific Crest Trail is a classic point-to-point hike (or winter ski tour) with great views from the ridge along the way. Celebrate your accomplishments with après-hike food and drink in the Village at Squaw Valley.

🚶🚶 From the parking lot at Sugar Bowl Academy, follow the small paved road on the west side of the parking lot. Head south to connect with the Overland Emigrant Trailhead in the Donner Summit area of the Tahoe National Forest.

From here the PCT ascends almost immediately through a small aspen grove via a handful of rocky switchbacks, revealing instant and awesome views of Donner Lake to the east. It then continues along a low ridgeline providing views of Mount Disney and the headwaters of the Yuba River, which looks like an enormous meadow to the northwest.

After about the first mile, a trail coming in from the left (east) heads toward Donner Summit. Stay right to begin the mellow ascent up to Roller Pass, where immigrants in the 1800s used roller logs to drive their oxen over the pass.

The trail wraps beneath Mount Lincoln offering plenty of views into Coldstream Valley, the town of Truckee and the airport, and a glimpse of Donner Lake. Some steep sections beneath Mount Lincoln can be snowed in late or early in the season. Be careful, as sections of the trail cut through steep, loose gullies.

N

0	1	2

miles

80

Pacific Crest Trail

Donner Pass Rd.

80

Norden

Donner Lake

Donner Pass Rd.

S. Yuba River

Overland Emigrant Trailhead

Donner Peak

Andover

Jackass Point

Mt. Judah

Crows Nest

Mt. Disney

Roller Pass Historic Area

TAHOE NATIONAL FOREST

Mt. Lincoln

Pacific Crest Trail

Cold Creek

Cedar Creek

S. Fork Cold Creek

Benson Hut

Anderson Peak

Coldstream Trail

Deep Creek

N. Fork American River

Tinker Knob

Billys Peak

Pole Creek

Painted Rock

Painted Rock Trail

Chief Creek

Silver Peak

Lyon Peak

Needle Peak

Granite Chief

Granite Chief Trail

Squaw Creek

Olympic Village Inn

Squaw Valley Rd.

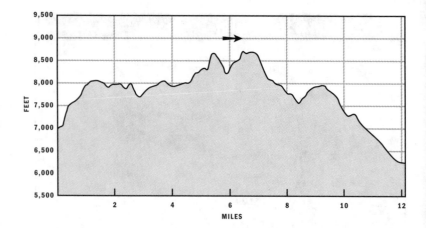

After this, the trail becomes incredibly easy for awhile, descending a gentle slope covered in mule's ears. Just shy of 4 miles, views of the Royal Gorge to the west begin replacing views to the east as the trail drops below the ridge. In about another mile, you'll notice a couple of out-of-place volcanic spires marking a trail passage.

Shortly after, the trail splits. Keep right to continue on the PCT. The trail left up the ridge leads to the Benson Hut, maintained by the Sierra Club. The hut sleeps 12 and stays warm with a wood-burning stove; bedding and food is not provided. The hut is more popular in the winter than in the summer, but reservations ($15 per person per night) are necessary year-round, call (800) 679-6775 or visit www.ctl.sierraclub.org for details.

The PCT proper cuts beneath the Benson Hut, about 0.5 miles farther south, and continues over a very rocky talus run-out. Shortly after the talus field, a cross pointing to Anderson Peak marks a beautiful view of the North Fork of the American River canyon to the west. Around the back side of Anderson Peak the trail becomes dusty,

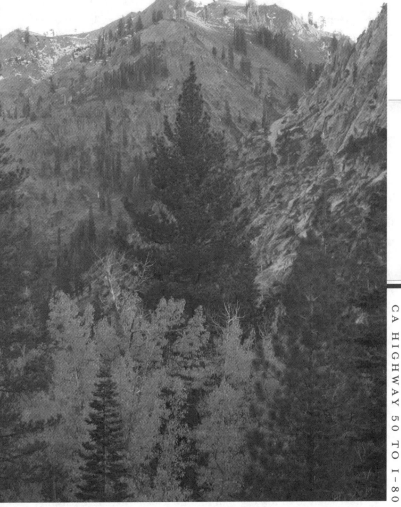

Granite Chief is part of Squaw Valley USA, home of the 1960 Winter Olympics.

with a steep drop-off; be careful. Views into Granite Chief and the Desolation wildernesses begin to open up.

The first glimpse of Lake Tahoe comes just before mile 7. At exactly mile 7 the trail splits again. A right turn takes you to Tinker Knob (elevation 8,949). Keep left to continue on the PCT and you'll notice another juncture in less than a half mile with the 15E05 trail leading into Coldstream Canyon.

Continue on the PCT, which begins dropping into the lush back bowls behind Tinker Knob and into the headwaters of the North Fork of the American River. At mile 8.3 there's a stream crossing, which makes a good water stop if you've packed a filter. This is hands down the prettiest part of the trail thus far, pines framing high-mountain views while you travel beneath a spiny ridgeline.

The rock also begins shifting to reveal granite boulder gardens. Leading into a dense conifer forest, you reach a low point cross-ing the North Fork of the American River and a sign reassuring you that Squaw Valley is only another 4 miles away. It's correct, but in another mile there's another sign saying the same thing!

At mile 10.2, an unmarked trail (which is the Painted Rock Trail leading deep into the canyon) comes in from the right. Follow the trail left to continue toward Squaw. And finally, in just another mile, take a left turn onto the Granite Chief Trail.

Keep to the left on the granite slab next to the cliffs. Views of Squaw Valley Ski Resort, its gondola, and, of course, Lake Tahoe begin opening up. At mile 12.7 there's a stream crossing, and 1 mile farther you follow the trail to the right to access Olympic Village. The trail follows a rambling creek ensconced in a tiny aspen grove. A maze of trails crisscross the place, but just keep going downhill—from here all roads lead to Squaw.

Bear right to follow the trail into the Chamonix Place parking lot. Follow the parking lot to the left to reach the Olympic Village Inn. This is a good place to park the shuttle vehicle.

Take advantage of the amenities at the Village at Squaw to curb your après-hiking hunger. The village is on the south side of the enormous parking lot in the middle of the valley. Scope it out when you set the shuttle. In the village, you can find good pizza at Fireside Pizza and tasty comfort food plus good brew at Auld Dubliner.

DIRECTIONS   TO SUGAR BOWL ACADEMY PARKING LOT: From Sacramento, follow Interstate 80 east toward Truckee and exit at Norden/Soda Springs. Turn right on Old US 40 and continue 3.6 miles. The parking lot is on the right immediately after the turn to Sugar Bowl Ski Resort and before Donner Summit. From Truckee, follow Donner Pass Road to Donner Summit. The parking lot is on the left just after the summit.

TO SQUAW VALLEY: From I-80 at Norden/Soda Springs, continue eastbound toward Truckee. Exit at Truckee onto CA 89 South toward Lake Tahoe/Tahoe City/Squaw Valley. Follow CA 89 south 8 miles to the Squaw Valley Road. Turn right and follow Squaw Valley Road to the base of the mountain. Continue straight ahead at the 90-degree turn to set a shuttle vehicle in the Chamonix Place parking lot. And take a few minutes to familiarize yourself with the village prior to starting your hike so you have a plan après hike.

GPS Trailhead Coordinates	17 Sugar Bowl to Squaw Valley
UTM Zone (WGS 84)	10S
Easting	0730432
Northing	4355107
Latitude	N39° 18.8820′
Longitude	W120° 19.6310′

18 Glacier Meadows Trail to Donner Pass Road

SCENERY: ✿ ✿ ✿	DISTANCE: 7 miles round-trip
TRAIL CONDITION: ✿ ✿ ✿ ✿ ✿	HIKING TIME: 2–3 hours
CHILDREN: ✿ ✿ ✿ ✿ ✿	MAP: Trails Illustrated Tahoe National
DIFFICULTY: ✿	Forest
SOLITUDE: ✿	OUTSTANDING FEATURES: *Incredible acces-*
DOGS: ✿ ✿ ✿ ✿ ✿	*sibility, great views of Sierra's glaciated history, views of Donner Lake and Castle Peak*

This easily accessible, short out-and-back jaunt makes a perfect quick getaway. Starting from a bustling Interstate 80 rest area, hikers take a trip through geologic history on the Pacific Crest Trail overlooking Donner Lake. The trail crosses Donner Pass Road 3.6 miles from the freeway, which makes for a nice turnaround. To shorten the 7-mile hike, set up a shuttle vehicle in the Sugar Bowl Academy parking lot at the turnaround.

🚶🚶 This highly trafficked hike begins on a half-mile rest-area trail called the Glacier Meadows Trail. Pick up the interpretive trail east of the A-frame bathroom structure for the fastest access to the PCT.

The trail parallels the freeway to start but quickly ducks into towering fir forest. You'll pass three of the ten interpretive signs before connecting to the PCT. After 500 feet or so, veer left at the Y to continue on the Donner Rim Trail. The trail is really well marked with self-explanatory signs at every juncture. After a picturesque shallow lake on the right, the trail feeds into the PCT.

For this short trip, turn right toward Donner Pass and Mount Judah. The sign indicates that Donner Pass is 4 miles away. I clocked the mileage at 3.6, with little more than 250 feet in elevation gain on each leg, making this section perfect for beginners or children needing to unleash pent up road-trip energy. For the seasoned hiker,

18 Glacier Meadows Trail to Donner Pass Road

N
0
0.2
0.4
mile
Pacific Crest Trail
80
80
Glacier Meadows Trailhead
To Truckee
Donner Creek
Azalea Lake
Flora Lake
Pacific Crest Trail
TAHOE NATIONAL FOREST
To Truckee and Donner Lake
highest point
George R. Stewart Peak
Lytton Lake Rd.
Lake Angela
PRIVATE LAND
Lake Azalea Rd.
Donner Pass Rd.
Donner Pass Rd.
McGlashan Point
To 80
Pacific Crest Trail
Lake Mary

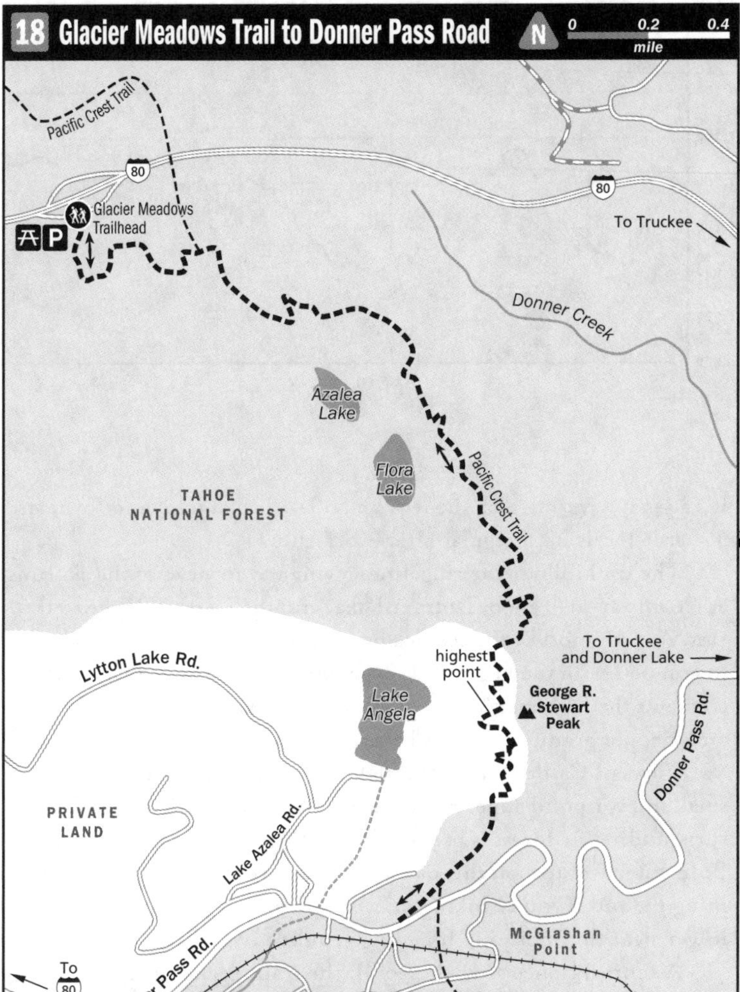

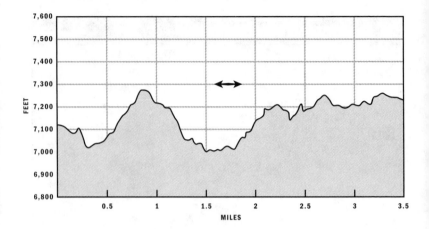

it's a great way to stretch the legs on an I-80 road trip, and for many Truckee locals it's a regular after-work run.

The trail follows the ridgeline, giving way to views of the ski runs at Northstar-at-Tahoe, Donner Lake, and the Carson Range to the east. As with most of the scenic appeal of this trail, every view seems to compete with the blight of I-80 rumbling in the distance. The trail cuts through manicured manzanita, huckleberry oak, and salt-and-pepper granite boulders before beginning a gradual climb.

Views of Castle Peak to the right open up and, shortly after, a small mirror pond appears on the left. While the reflection of the surrounding fir forest is beautiful, don't expect to go for a swim. Both water features on this particular trail are too shallow for swimming in, and if you're hiking in early spring you may not want to linger near this mosquito breeding ground.

A short distance after the pond, the trail reaches its crest. Here, take in a great look at the scope of Sugar Bowl Ski Resort and the top of Donner Ski Ranch directly in front of you. This area is very popu-

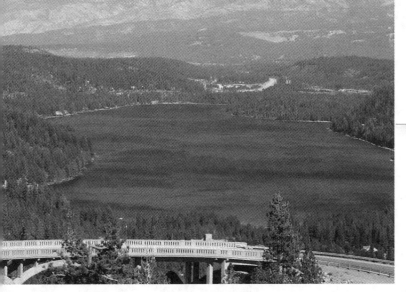

Expect views of Old Highway 40, Donner Lake, and the town of Truckee from the PCT.

lar for skiing in winter and rock climbing during the rest of the year. Don't be surprised if you see folks clinging to the black and gray–streaked granite cliffs that you'll pass on the descent toward Donner Pass Road.

The trail, which tops out around 7,250 feet, loses elevation quickly as it cuts a handful of switchbacks through lush manzanita shrubs. Less than a mile later you reach the turnaround point. There, look across the street for the Sugar Bowl Ski Academy. The building is the year-round training center for some of the next generation's world-class skiers, but don't expect to be able to use the restroom—a sign indicates that no public restrooms are available.

The views heading back are far better, since you'll be facing Donner Lake. You'll know you're getting close to the end when the rumble of I-80 picks up. This time, turn left at the first Y and left at the second Y to finish the interpretive trail. The first sign you come to provides an interesting look at a glacier-polished granite slab littered with erratic boulders. Pass the six remaining signs and come to one more Y before reaching the parking lot. Veer right at the last Y to finish the trail refreshed and ready for the drive ahead.

DIRECTIONS From Sacramento, follow I-80 east toward Reno. Exit at the rest area immediately past the Boreal/Pacific Crest Trailhead exit. From Reno, follow I-80 west toward Sacramento 45 miles. Exit at the rest area near the crest of Donner Summit 3.2 miles past the second Donner Lake exit.

GPS Trailhead Coordinates	18 Glacier Meadows Trail to Donner Pass Road
UTM Zone (WGS 84)	10S
Easting	0728397
Northing	4358741
Latitude	N39° 20.8770′
Longitude	W120° 20.9720′

Hiking north on the PCT from Old Highway 40 provides excellent views of Castle Peak.

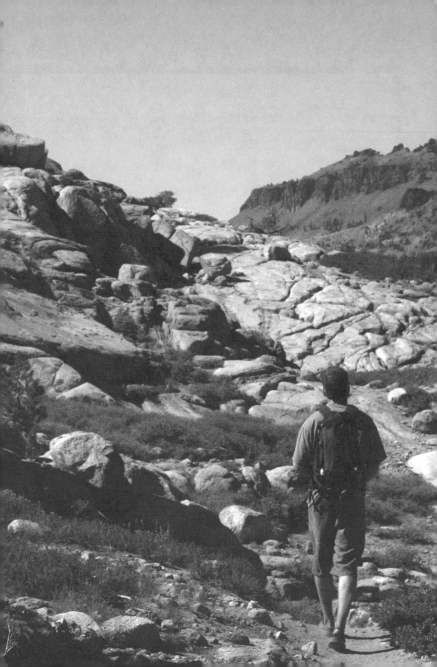

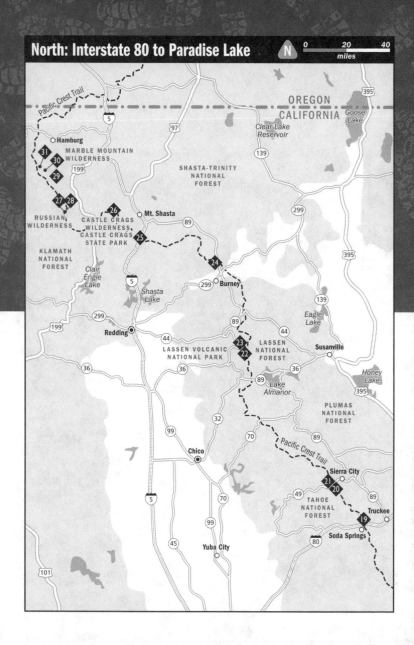

N

0   20   40
miles

OREGON
CALIFORNIA

Goose
Lake

395

5

97

Clear Lake
Reservoir

139

Hamburg

MARBLE MOUNTAIN
WILDERNESS

SHASTA-TRINITY
NATIONAL
FOREST

31

30

29

199

299

27   28

RUSSIAN
WILDERNESS

CASTLE CRAGS
WILDERNESS,
CASTLE CRAGS
STATE PARK

26

Mt. Shasta

25

89

KLAMATH
NATIONAL
FOREST

Clair
Engle
Lake

24

395

5

Shasta
Lake

299   Burney

199

299

Redding

44

Eagle
Lake

89

44

139

23

LASSEN
VOLCANIC
NATIONAL PARK

22

LASSEN
NATIONAL
FOREST

Susanville

36

36

36

Honey
Lake

395

89

Lake
Almanor

32

PLUMAS
NATIONAL
FOREST

99

70

89

Chico

Pacific Crest Trail

70

Sierra City

21   20

49

89

5

99

TAHOE
NATIONAL
FOREST

19

Truckee

Soda Springs

45

80

Yuba City

101

Pacific Crest Trail

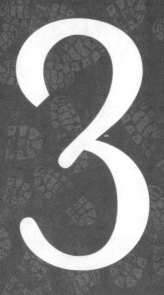

NORTH

Interstate 80 to
Paradise Lake

19 Warren Lake

SCENERY: ☆ ☆ ☆ ☆ ☆	HIKING TIME: *2 days*
TRAIL CONDITION: ☆ ☆ ☆	MAP: Trails Illustrated Tahoe National
CHILDREN: ☆ ☆	Forest
DIFFICULTY: ☆ ☆ ☆ ☆ ☆	OUTSTANDING FEATURES: *Excellent camping*
SOLITUDE: ☆ ☆ ☆	*and swimming at Warren Lake, great swimming at*
DISTANCE: *17 miles round-trip*	*Paradise Lake, beautiful wildflowers in summer*

This excellent weekend loop hike on the Pacific Crest and Warren Lake trails includes incredible camping on Warren Lake, excellent swimming at both Warren and Paradise lakes, and fields of wildflowers all the way there and back.

🚶 Follow Andesite Ridge Road from Interstate 80. Turn right on the first double-track road to connect to the PCT as it climbs through Castle Valley below Castle Peak's southwest face. You can also access the PCT directly from the rest area on the north side of I-80. Either way, in about 4 miles you reach Castle Pass where the PCT connects with Andesite Ridge Road and, shortly after, an unmaintained trail following the ridge northeast to Castle Peak. Continue north (staying slightly left) on the PCT and drop into the beautiful, lush Round Valley where Castle Creek drenches the valley before draining into the South Yuba River Canyon to the west.

Follow the PCT—crossing a tangled path of running water—across the meadow. You might notice a small cabin left of the PCT set back in the trees. This is the Peter Grubb Hut, a backcountry shelter maintained by the Sierra Club. The hut is more popular in the winter with backcountry skiers, than in the summer with hikers but reservations ($15 per person, per night) can be made year-round, call (800) 679-6775 or visit www.ctl.sierraclub.org for details.

Near the north end of the meadow, a well-traveled trail turns to the left (west) and heads out toward Fordyce Lake. Continue on the PCT following the sign toward Paradise Creek (directly north). The PCT steadily climbs away from Round Valley, leaving views of Castle

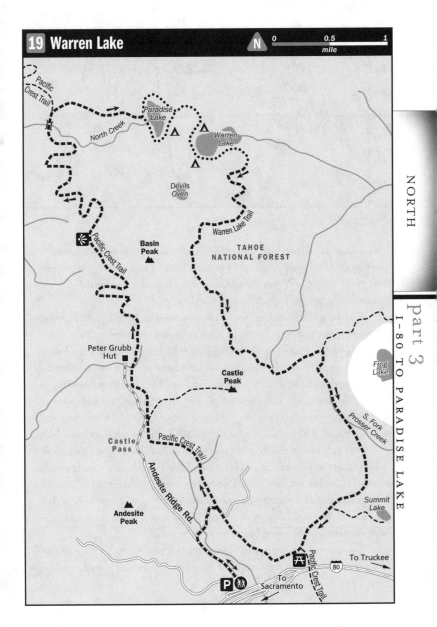

N

0   0.5   1
mile

Pacific Crest Trail

Paradise Lake

North Creek

Warren Lake

Devils Oven

Pacific Crest Trail

Basin Peak

Warren Lake Trail

TAHOE NATIONAL FOREST

NORTH

Peter Grubb Hut

Castle Peak

part 3
I-80 TO PARADISE LAKE

Frog Lake

S. Fork Prosser Creek

Castle Pass

Pacific Crest Trail

Andesite Ridge Rd.

Andesite Peak

Summit Lake

To Sacramento

Pacific Crest Trail

80

To Truckee

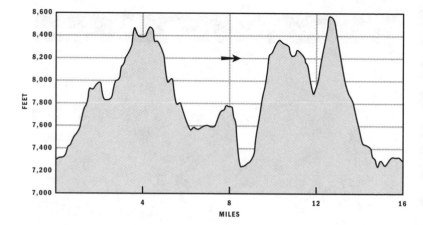

Peak, Round Valley, and Granite Chief Wilderness in the distance at your back. The trail contours beneath Basin Peak, providing excellent views into the Yuba River Canyon before dropping steeply into dense forest on its way to Paradise Valley.

Within a few hundred yards of crossing the nice footbridge spanning the slow-moving Paradise Creek, look for a trail to Paradise Lake off to the right (east). Here, you split from the PCT and continue on the off-road-vehicle trail, climbing steadily over polished granite bedrock, boulders, and marsh, before reaching Paradise Lake. Paradise Lake is a great swimming and fishing lake with excellent sloping granite cliffs for jumping off into the lake on the southwest side and a handful of nice campsites scattered around the lake.

You can circle the lake on its north side following a faint trail (overgrown in places) or circle around the south side, which requires a bit of boulder scrambling. The north route is easier. Head for the low, granite saddle on the far-east side, where you'll catch your first glimpse of Warren Lake, a beautiful lake sunken into the landscape beneath steep cliffs on at least three of its sides.

If you have the luxury of spending two nights out, camp above Warren Lake on the first night. The perfect summer evening is spent

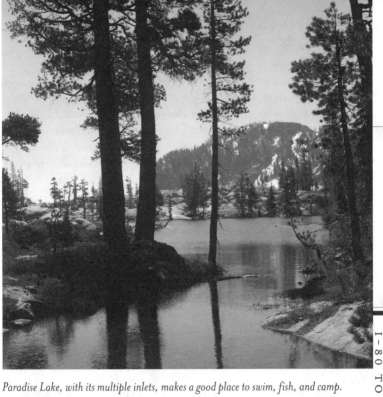

Paradise Lake, with its multiple inlets, makes a good place to swim, fish, and camp.

watching the sunset over Paradise Lake and then waking as the sun rises over Warren Lake.

Descending to Warren Lake is a bit tricky and will take some confidence in traveling off-trail. The best way down is heading slightly north from the saddle. Although there is a bit of bushwhacking involved, there aren't any impassable cliff bands to negotiate. Some maps show a trail leading from Paradise Lake to Warren Lake, but I never found anything that qualified as a definite trail.

It's easy to see where the lake is, and heading carefully downhill toward it will get you there in no time. Once at lake level, you'll find the best camping around the south and southwest side of the lake where

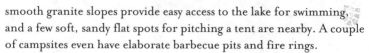

smooth granite slopes provide easy access to the lake for swimming, and a few soft, sandy flat spots for pitching a tent are nearby. A couple of campsites even have elaborate barbecue pits and fire rings.

To leave Warren Lake and continue on the loop hike via Warren Lake Trail, follow the shoreline to the south side of Warren Lake. As you enter a wooded area along the lake keep an eye out for a developed campsite with a prominent fire ring. Directly behind the campsite a sign posted to a tree reads WARREN LAKE and a trail immediately ascending. The Warren Lake Trail, ascending near the sign, can be tricky to find. Avoid the urge to turn up the unnamed creek bed early and remember that the trail follows the creek on its east (left) side as it climbs steeply to the bowls behind Castle and Basin peaks.

Once you've crested, it's easy to see the way out. The trail hugs a contour line in about the middle of Castle Peak's back side bowl, through lush wildflower fields before it climbs again to the back side of Frog Lake Cliffs. Continue south, descending steadily through thick forest toward I-80. Approximately 1 mile from the freeway is a trail leading 0.5 miles to Summit Lake. Follow the Warren Lake Trail to its intersection with the PCT to complete this loop.

DIRECTIONS From I-80, exit at Castle Peak/Boreal and continue to a dirt parking lot on the north side of the freeway. Additional parking is available on the south side of the freeway. The PCT heading north can also be accessed only from I-80 westbound.

PERMITS Overnight users are advised to pick up a fire permit from any ranger station or Cal Fire station.

GPS Trailhead Coordinates	19 Warren Lake
UTM Zone (WGS 84)	10S
Easting	0728591
Northing	4357990
Latitude	N39° 20.8756′
Longitude	W120° 20.9143′

20 Loves Falls

SCENERY: ⛏ ⛏ ⛏
TRAIL CONDITION: ⛏ ⛏ ⛏ ⛏ ⛏
CHILDREN: ⛏ ⛏ ⛏ ⛏ ⛏
DIFFICULTY: ⛏
SOLITUDE: ⛏ ⛏

DISTANCE: *1 mile round-trip (or alternate 5 miles round-trip)*
HIKING TIME: *1–2 hours*
MAP: Trails Illustrated Tahoe National Forest
OUTSTANDING FEATURES: *Loves Falls, views of Sierra Buttes*

Loves Falls makes a pretty destination on the Pacific Crest Trail. Access the PCT directly from CA 49 for a quick 1-mile round-trip hike, or start on the Wild Plum Loop for a longer, 5-mile round-trip.

🧍🧍 Loves Falls is very easily accessed from CA 49. Simply pull off the highway at the sign where the PCT crosses the road, and follow the PCT downhill (south) for about 0.5 miles to the falls. If your priority is seeing waterfalls for the day, that's the best way to access them.

For a longer route and a nice afternoon hike or trail run to Loves Falls, start from the Wild Plum Trailhead parking lot on Wild Plum Road. From the lot, follow the trail past the outhouse restrooms and down to Haypress Creek. The trail quickly crosses Wild Plum Road at the bridge over Haypress Creek. A sign at this intersection directs foot traffic in the same direction for the Wild Plum Loop, Haypress Trail, and the PCT. Hike along the creek bed for less than 1 mile through cedar forest, climbing a moderate, winding grade to the intersection with the PCT.

At the intersection, follow the trail to the left (north). From here, Loves Falls is approximately 1 mile away. The trail follows the ridge, cutting into some rocky switchbacks that provide great views of the Sierra Buttes and the North Fork of the Yuba River canyon.

This hike is a great outing for families and dogs, but locals warn that rattlesnakes like to curl up on the trail, especially in spring and summer, so use caution. If you are coming from Wild Plum

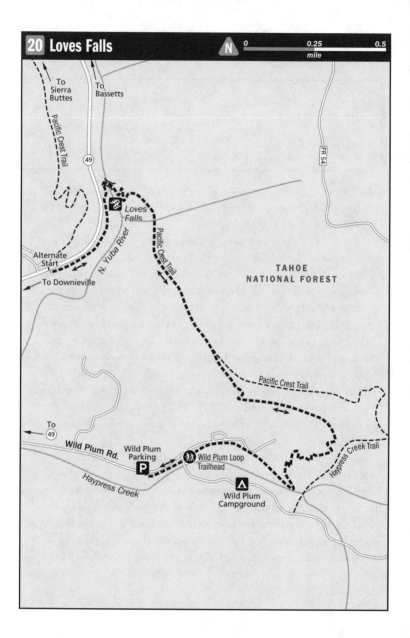

N

0   0.25   0.5
            mile

To
Sierra
Buttes

To
Bassetts

Pacific Crest Trail

49

Loves
Falls

Pacific Crest Trail

N. Yuba River

Alternate
Start

To Downieville

FR 54

TAHOE
NATIONAL FOREST

Pacific Crest Trail

To
49

Wild Plum Rd.

Wild Plum
Parking

P

Wild Plum Loop
Trailhead

Wild Plum
Campground

Haypress Creek

Haypress Creek Trail

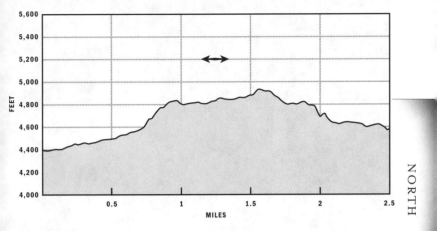

Campground, you will see one trickling stream crossing just before you reach the falls.

An arched bridge crosses the North Yuba River above Loves Falls. Upstream of the bridge, the river canyon is dramatic and narrow. Below Loves Falls is a nice-sized pool that can be good for a quick dip. Be careful, however, not to be swept away—there is another waterfall just downstream of the bridge. This lower waterfall is the more dramatic of the two; it's nice to spend the afternoon lying on the smooth granite boulders overlooking the falls. There'll be no swimming here, though, as after the waterfall the canyon becomes a gorge.

This hike, which averages around 4,600 feet in elevation for its entirety, is best done in the late spring and early summer, when the river is full of water. The falls often dry up by early fall.

part 3
I-80 TO PARADISE LAKE

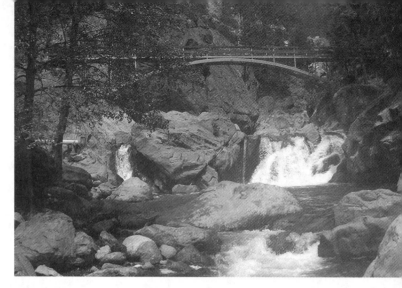

Loves Falls drops 12 feet on the North Yuba River.

DIRECTIONS From Downieville, follow CA 49 north 13 miles. Turn right onto Wild Plum Road and follow it 1.2 miles to access the trailhead parking. Traveling south on CA 49 from Bassetts, go 4.5 miles before turning left onto Wild Plum Road. The PCT crosses CA 49 exactly 3.8 miles south of Bassetts or 14 miles north of Downieville.

GPS Trailhead Coordinates	20 Loves Falls
UTM Zone (WGS 84)	10S
Easting	0705899
Northing	4382491
Latitude	N39° 34.0453'
Longitude	W120° 36.1835'

21 Sierra Buttes Lookout

SCENERY: ✰ ✰ ✰ ✰ ✰	DISTANCE: *5.2 miles round-trip*
TRAIL CONDITION: ✰ ✰ ✰ ✰ ✰	HIKING TIME: *2–4 hours*
CHILDREN: ✰ ✰ ✰ ✰ ✰	MAP: Trails Illustrated Tahoe National
DIFFICULTY: ✰ ✰	Forest
SOLITUDE: ✰	OUTSTANDING FEATURES: *Incredible views,*
DOGS: ✰ ✰ ✰ ✰ ✰	*abandoned fire lookout*

This popular short hike accesses one of the most remarkable views in Northern California.

👫 Everybody and their brother, mother, and grandmother hikes up to the abandoned fire lookout on the top of the Sierra Buttes, but that isn't necessarily because it's easy. No matter how you go—and there are at least three different routes—it's a steady and steep climb to the top. But it's worth it. And that's why, if you're looking for a quick shot of inspiration in the form of spectacular 360-degree views of Northern California's diverse landscape, this is the place to go. Mind you, if you're squeamish about off-road vehicle traffic marring the hiking experience, you should start early in the morning on an off-season weekday.

Of the three routes to the top, there's a long, hot route along the Pacific Crest Trail heading north that starts at CA 49; an extremely short route following only the jeep trail to the top; and a 5.2-mile out-and-back version that splits the difference and offers some beautiful lake views and singletrack hiking along the way.

My advice is to pursue the latter, and here's how: The Pacific Crest Trail, marked 12E06, starts off as a wide path through a green metal gate. After about 0.5 miles of climbing, the road narrows to a singletrack trail toward the right. Follow the singletrack for 0.3 miles as it runs along the ridge offering views of the Sutter Buttes to the west and the Sierra Buttes to the southeast.

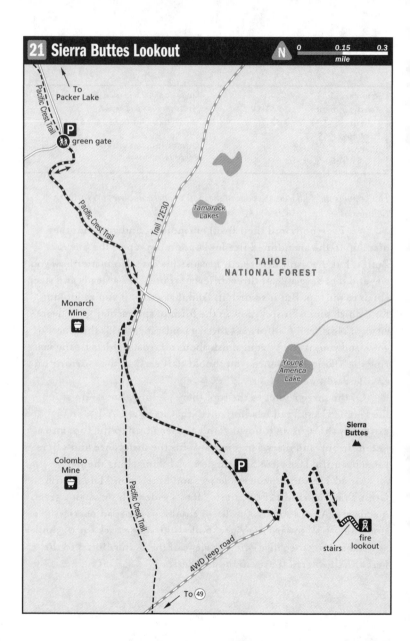

N

0   0.15   0.3
mile

To
Packer Lake

Pacific Crest Trail

P

green gate

Pacific Crest Trail

Trail 12E30

Tamarack
Lakes

TAHOE
NATIONAL FOREST

Monarch
Mine

Young
America
Lake

Colombo
Mine

Sierra
Buttes

P

Pacific Crest Trail

stairs

fire
lookout

4WD jeep road

To 49

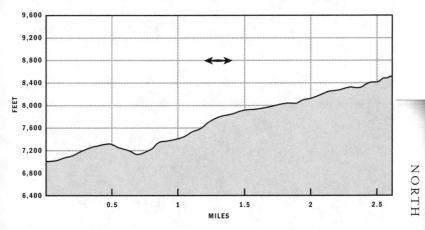

Just before the first mile, the PCT veers to the right (southwest) and begins descending toward Loves Falls around the south base of the Buttes. Stay left (slightly southeast), to access the Butte summit on the Tamarack Connector Trail 12E30. After this, continue straight on the main path and walk along the ridgeline, as a few trails will criss-cross this route along the way. The view of Young America Lake lying almost 2,000 near-vertical feet beneath the pinnacle of the Sierra Buttes is quite something, and there are smooth boulders to sit on and take in the scenery.

The trail ducks into a small forest dotted with enormous rusty-colored boulders before coming to a small parking area, unpaved and accessed by a 4WD-only road, at mile 1.6. This junction I marked at mile 1.6. The trail picks up again on the opposite side of the parking area, and at mile 1.8 it hooks up with a jeep road. Although many hikers complain about 4WD vehicles whizzing past them on the trail, I've never experienced such annoyances.

Time this hike for a weekday morning in the late autumn when a dusting of fresh snow decorates the distant peaks of Mount Rose and

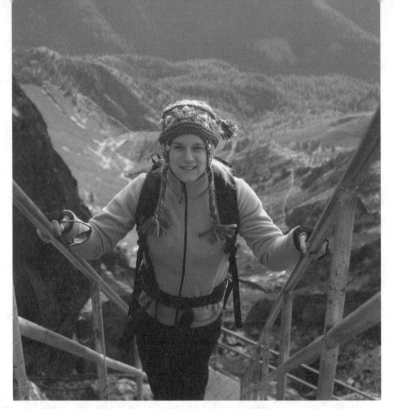

Three steep, steel staircases lead to the top of the Sierra Buttes fire lookout where the views are worth the work.

a number of peaks in Desolation Wilderness when the views are the best and traffic least likely. Views of the heavily forested canyon wilderness to the north and west are incredible from the jeep road (at any time of year) and keep getting better toward the top.

The route becomes increasingly steep before reaching the infamous metal stairs, which climb the last 100 feet in elevation to the 8,598-foot summit in approximately 300 feet.

While you're climbing this stairway to heaven of sorts, thank the five Tahoe National Forest employees who hauled the materials to build the lookout in 1964. Another interesting thought to keep your mind off the clear drop-off or the climb is the incredible geologic conception of the Buttes. Born out of an undersea volcanic eruption an estimated 350 million years ago, this giant sentinel is resistant to erosion and a miner's jackpot. In 1869, some lucky soul found a 106-pound nugget at the Monumental Mine near the Buttes, and by the early 1900s 11 mines were operating on or near the Buttes. Although the mines and the gold are gone today, from the top of the fire lookout you'll still think you've found your fortune.

DIRECTIONS   From Sacramento, take Interstate 80 east to Auburn. Exit CA 49 north toward Nevada City. Continue northeast through Sierra City and turn left on the Gold Lake Highway at Bassets. Go 1.4 miles before turning left onto Packer Lake Road.

In 0.5 miles take a right toward Packer Lake and Deer Lake Trail. Continue left on National Forest Road 93, passing a sign to the Tamarack Lakes Trailhead and a PCT trailhead toward Gold Lakes.

Approximately 0.5 miles after the first PCT trailhead sign, you'll see another PCT trailhead sign on the left. This is the beginning of the hike. Limited parking is available at the gate.

GPS Trailhead Coordinates	21 Sierra Buttes Lookout
UTM Zone (WGS 84)	10S
Easting	0700426
Northing	4387254
Latitude	N39° 36.696'
Longitude	W120° 39.917'

22 Warner Valley Road to Terminal Geyser

SCENERY: ✿ ✿	HIKING TIME: *2–3 hours*
TRAIL CONDITION: ✿ ✿ ✿ ✿	MAP: Lassen Volcanic National Park *by*
CHILDREN: ✿ ✿ ✿ ✿ ✿	*Wilderness Press*
DIFFICULTY: ✿	OUTSTANDING FEATURES: *Boiling Springs*
SOLITUDE: ✿ ✿ ✿	*Lake, Terminal Geyser, flowery hillsides in spring*
DISTANCE: *5.4 miles round-trip*	

Terminal Geyser is one of the few easily accessible geothermal features on the Pacific Crest Trail and a worthy destination for this relatively easy loop hike in Lassen Volcanic National Park.

🏃 Lassen Volcanic National Park's off-the-beaten-path location offers superb hiking and fascinating geothermal features, such as the Sulphur Works system—an underground furnace with five chimneys.

This hike joins the PCT for a short while and leads to one of the noisiest escape routes of these scalding subterranean waters. The geyser is a delightfully eerie destination on this out-and-back or loop hike and a great one for kids—scientific and geologic lessons abound.

Timing the trip to Terminal Geyser should be done with care; late spring or early fall are best. Too early in the spring or too late in the fall expect a road closure 2.5 miles from the trailhead, which adds an extra 5 miles of walking on Warner Valley Road paralleling Hot Springs Creek. Call the park at (530) 595-4480 to check for closures.

The bonus to making the trip after the road has closed is the solitude. Most folks go only as far as Boiling Springs Lake—a smoking, gray pond that stays at around 125°F. Students from nearby Chico State University use the highly acidic pond as an outdoor biological research lab.

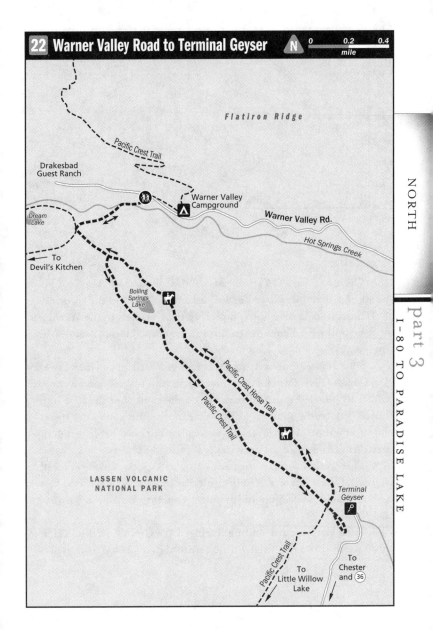

Flatiron Ridge

Pacific Crest Trail

Drakesbad
Guest Ranch

Warner Valley
Campground

Warner Valley Rd.

Hot Springs Creek

Dream
Lake

← To
Devil's Kitchen

Boiling
Springs
Lake

Pacific Crest Horse Trail

Pacific Crest Trail

LASSEN VOLCANIC
NATIONAL PARK

Terminal
Geyser

Pacific Crest Trail

To
Little Willow
Lake

To
Chester
and 36

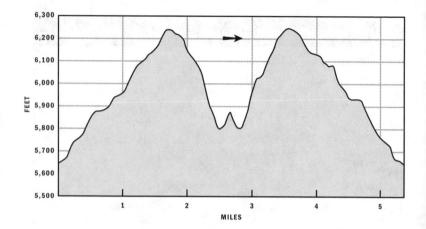

There are two PCT trailheads off the access road. The first heads
north to Corral Meadow. For this hike, turn left into the second
PCT trailhead parking lot and pick up the trail next to the Warner
Valley Trail sign. From the trailhead, Terminal Geyser is 2.7 miles
one-way.

Shortly after the start, a trail bridge crosses Hot Springs Creek.
Drakesbad Guest Ranch and cabins come into full view and a couple
of faintly traveled spur trails appear on the right after the first 0.3
miles. Taking the spur trails might mean you find your soles steaming after a short while. Warnings are posted to keep hikers on designated trail areas and off potentially scalding hot spots.

This trail, although confusing in some spots, is also very well
signed. Take a left at the first sign pointing toward Terminal Geyser. At the second sign and juncture, go left to Boiling Springs
Lake.

Turn right toward Boiling Springs Lake Circuit on the PCT and
head south through a thick forest before arriving at a stream cross-

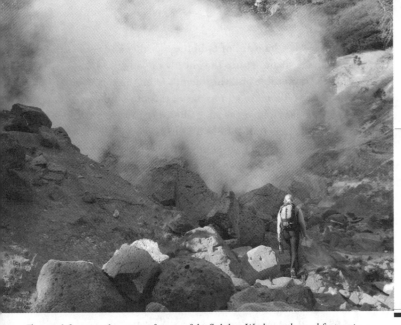

Terminal Geyser is the noisiest feature of the Sulphur Works geothermal feature in Lassen Volcanic National Park.

ing. Circumnavigate Boiling Springs Lake by going right or left; I prefer crossing the stream and heading right along the south side of the lake, where you'll find some of the best mud pots in the park.

Shortly after leaving the bubbling, steaming pit of gray-green water, the trail hooks up with the PCT again. At the junction, go right toward Terminal Geyser. Head right again at the next junction. Left leads to Little Willow Lake, which dries up in the fall and is a mosquito cesspool in early summer. Opt for the supernatural forces at Terminal Geyser instead.

You can hear the hiss and smell the sulfur long before reaching the feature. The trail descends a short, rocky hillside and then promptly turns up a canyon. At the end of the canyon you find the geyser—an impressive handful of bubbling puddles and vents shooting warm, sulfuric steam jets up the ghostly hillside.

The view is incredible and the warmth from the steam eases the chill on a cool day. To make a loop out of this out-and-back hike, on the way back bear right at the sign labeled PCT HORSE TRAIL in black marker pen. This trail follows a hillside covered in mule's ears instead of Boiling Springs Lake, but you can still see the steam rising through the forest on the way back. Make a right at each diversion and you'll find yourself back at the car.

DIRECTIONS From Red Bluff, follow CA 36 for 68.7 miles to Chester. In Chester, turn left on Warner Valley Road and continue 17 miles to the trailhead. Keep left at the first Y and right at the second Y.

PERMITS No permits are necessary for day use in this area. Camping is allowed in the Warner Valley Campground. Reservations can be made at www.recreation.gov.

GPS Trailhead Coordinates	22 Warner Valley Road to Terminal Geyser
UTM Zone (WGS 84)	10T
Easting	0635907
Northing	4478154
Latitude	N40° 26.5760'
Longitude	W121° 23.8480'

23 Cluster Lakes

SCENERY: ✿ ✿ ✿ ✿
TRAIL CONDITION: ✿ ✿ ✿ ✿ ✿
CHILDREN: ✿ ✿ ✿
(overnight ✿ ✿ ✿ ✿ ✿)
DIFFICULTY: ✿
SOLITUDE: ✿ ✿

NOTE: *Summer crowds swell, but visitor traffic to Lassen is the least of any national park in California.*
DISTANCE: *12.8 miles round-trip*
HIKING TIME: *4—8 hours*
MAP: Lassen Volcanic National Park *by Wilderness Press*
OUTSTANDING FEATURES: *Lots of small, wooded lakes and views of Lassen Peak*

Lake-loving hikers are bound to enjoy this 12.8-mile jaunt through the Cluster Lakes in Lassen Volcanic National Park. This hike also has the perfect gradient for trail running, which I highly recommend if you're up for it. Joining the Pacific Crest Trail for a mere mile, you'll find a wooded wonderland tucked into one of the least visited national parks.

🚶🚶 The Summit Lake Trailhead is well marked with a map sign at the start. Begin the hike by crossing the meadow bridge, and within a hundred yards you reach Summit Lake, a mirror for Lassen Peak and Brokeoff Mountain. The view is best from the east side of the lake, which is exactly the way you are heading—save your cameras for then.

After a third of a mile you come to a trail sign; take a left toward Echo Lake and begin a short climb on rocky soil into open dwarf forest while Lassen and Brokeoff mountains tower at your back. About 0.75 miles up the climb you reach the next junction. This is essentially where you begin the loop. Turn east toward Echo Lake to follow this guide.

About 0.75 miles from the junction you reach Echo Lake—a small, long lake with a beautiful milky-green color. The cluster has begun, and in less than another mile, at mile 2.7, you reach the next lake—a small pond with a steep north-facing slope. From here, there's a different lake about every half mile for almost the entire loop.

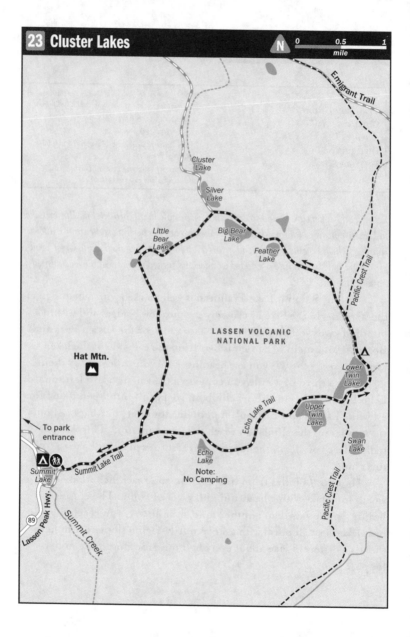

N

| 0 | 0.5 | 1 |

mile

Emigrant Trail

Cluster Lake

Silver Lake

Little Bear Lake

Big Bear Lake

Feather Lake

Pacific Crest Trail

LASSEN VOLCANIC NATIONAL PARK

Hat Mtn.

Lower Twin Lake

To park entrance

Echo Lake Trail

Upper Twin Lake

Swan Lake

Summit Lake Trail

Echo Lake

Note: No Camping

Summit Lake

89

Lassen Peak Hwy.

Summit Creek

Pacific Crest Trail

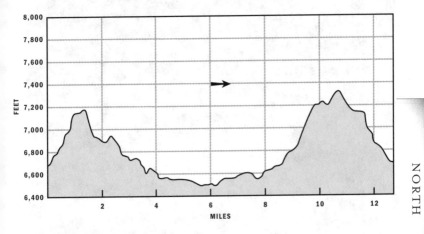

The trail is incredibly picturesque, hugging lake shoreline almost the entire time. After the first descent on the trail, you reach Lower Twin Lake, the largest of the group. At its southwest end a small stream from Upper Twin Lake (which you pass at mile 3.1) empties into its lower twin. At this juncture, hang right around the lake to hook up with the PCT at mile 4.4.

To circle the Cluster Lakes, make a left and head north. The PCT hugs Lower Twin Lake, traveling through a recently burned forest until reaching its northeastern edge, where there is an excellent camping beach and meadow with sunset views.

On the trail, keep left to follow the PCT west of Fairfield Peak. Soon after, veer off the PCT and head left toward Feather Lake to complete the Cluster circuit. The PCT continues directly north, while the trail to Feather Lake heads in a more northwesterly direction. Feather Lake is just as pretty as the rest, though probably not ideal for camping on the beach covered in lava rocks. Each lake in the circuit has its own unique quality, and exploring the lakes one after another is a memorable experience.

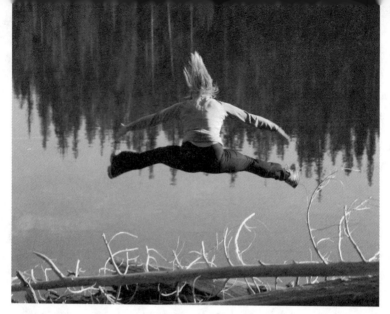

A hiker expresses her enthusiasm for placid, peaceful Silver Lake.

Silver Lake (where the camping is better) is next, less than 0.5 miles from Feather. Three quarters of a mile from Silver Lake, take a left at the trail juncture toward the Bear Lakes. The trail begins to climb past Little Bear Lake through dwarf forest, and at mile 8.7 your short climb is rewarded with a spectacular view of the volcanic Mount Hoffman and Prospect Peaks to the east. Look west to see Lassen Peak coming into view again also.

Traveling through the Jeffrey pine forest, the trail begins its descent and the views of Lassen Peak improve. Making the journey in late afternoon, you'll likely see incredible cloud colors near Lassen near sunset. As you descend, look for a faint spur trail leading to the right to get the best open view of Lassen before completing this spectacular loop hike.

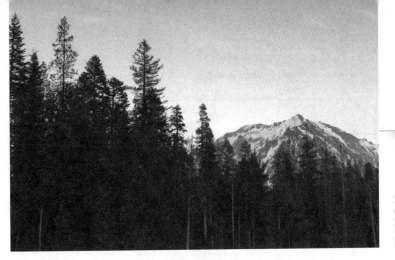

Views of Mount Lassen, the southernmost active volcano in the Cascade Range, are common from the Cluster Lakes circuit.

DIRECTIONS From Redding, travel east on CA 44 for 48 miles. Turn south onto CA 89 and drive 12 miles into Lassen Volcanic National Park. The park entrance fee is $10. From the park entrance, go 1.7 miles south into the park to the Summit Lake Ranger Station Trailhead. Turn left into the parking lot. Be aware that the park campgrounds generally close in the middle of September.

PERMITS Free wilderness permits are required to camp outside of designated campgrounds in Lassen Volcanic National Park. In this area, camping is prohibited around Echo Lake. Wilderness permits can be obtained in person at any contact station in the park during regular business hours or reserved online at www.nps.gov/lavo/planyourvisit. Reservations for Summit Lake North and Summit Lake South campgrounds can be made at www.recreation.gov.

GPS Trailhead Coordinates	23 Cluster Lakes
UTM Zone (WGS 84)	10T
Easting	0633298
Northing	4484201
Latitude	N40° 29.869′
Longitude	W121° 25.6160′

24 Burney Falls

SCENERY: ✿ ✿ ✿ ✿ ✿	DISTANCE: *2.7 miles round-trip*
TRAIL CONDITION: ✿ ✿ ✿ ✿ ✿	HIKING TIME: *1 hour*
CHILDREN: ✿ ✿ ✿ ✿ ✿	MAP: McArthur–Burney Falls Memorial
DIFFICULTY: ✿	State Park *by California State Parks*
SOLITUDE: ✿	OUTSTANDING FEATURES: *Burney Falls, great*
	trout fishing in Burney Creek

This easy but scenic hike is a great leg stretcher early in the hiking season, when many of the Pacific Crest Trail's other sections are under snow. At just under 3,000 feet for the entire length of the hike, this area comes alive in springtime with birdsong and blossoms. The falls are a wonder to behold as well.

🚶🚶 The highlight of the hike is no doubt Burney Falls, where 100 million gallons of beautiful, milky-blue water drop 129 feet over a near-vertical basaltic lava ledge. Watch Burney Creek burst to life as it's fed by thousands of underground streams by starting your hike on the PCT at the trailhead on Clark Creek Road. Turn right (south toward Mexico 1,418 miles away) and follow the PCT less than 1 mile toward Headwaters Camp, where you'll find a picnic area with restrooms, picnic tables, and a corral.

Shortly after the camp, the PCT crosses Burney Creek on a small footbridge. Pay special attention to the creek at this point in the hike—it's barely flowing! Pointing this out to children (of all ages) is a great way to illustrate the evidence of the creek's underground springs as the creek character changes dramatically downstream.

Shortly after crossing the creek, bear left on the Headwaters Trail (toward Burney Falls). The trail follows the creek bed through black and white oak trees, the occasional vine maple, and vibrant, purple deer brush.

As the trail becomes paved, hug the railing past the interpretive sign, following the paved switchbacks through a towering incense cedar stand to the foot of the falls. If it's a hot day, you'll be tempted

136

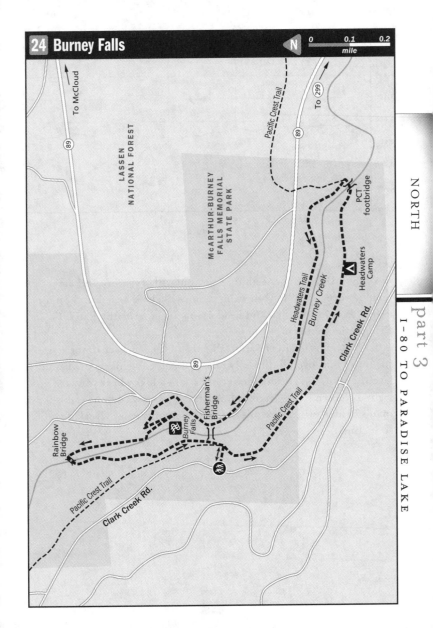

To McCloud

89

LASSEN
NATIONAL
FOREST

Pacific Crest Trail

89

To 299

PCT
footbridge

McARTHUR-BURNEY
FALLS MEMORIAL
STATE PARK

Headwaters Trail

Burney Creek

Headwaters
Camp

Clark Creek Rd.

89

Fisherman's
Bridge

Pacific Crest Trail

Rainbow
Bridge

Burney
Falls

Pacific Crest Trail

Clark Creek Rd.

NORTH

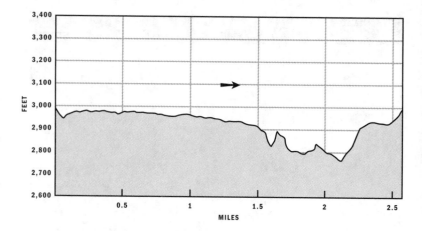

to swim in the pool beneath the falls, but with a year-round water temperature of 48°F, your swim is more likely to be a dip. Stop for awhile to enjoy the view and head downstream, crossing Rainbow Bridge (the first bridge you see).

The trail gains in elevation slightly on the way back to the starting point but, overall, this easy hike is suitable for hikers of all ability levels. Follow the Headwaters Trail back to a fork where you take a right to return to the trailhead. A left takes a short detour to Fisherman's Bridge, which provides a scenic view of Burney Creek if you're so inclined.

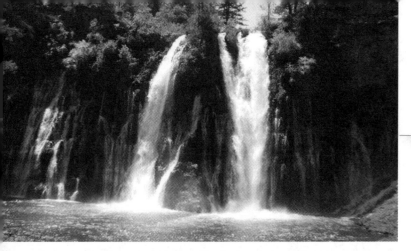

More than 100 million gallons of water falls 129 feet year-round at Burney Falls.

DIRECTIONS From the intersection of CA 44 and CA 89, travel north on CA 89 for 26 miles. Turn left onto Clark Creek Road and follow it 1.7 miles. There is an unpaved trailhead parking lot on the right. There are no restrooms at this trailhead.

From Redding, travel east on CA 299 to its intersection with CA 89 and bear left (north) 4.2 miles before turning left onto Clark Creek Road. Traveling south on CA 89 from Interstate 5, follow CA 89 for 52.2 miles before making a right onto Clark Creek Road, 0.5 miles past the McArthur-Burney Falls Falls State Park entrance.

Hikers can also access this trail from inside McArthur-Burney Falls Memorial State Park; the park entrance fee is $10.

PERMITS No permits are necessary for day use on this trail. Camping and cabin rental is available inside the state park. More information is available at www.parks.ca.gov.

GPS Trailhead Coordinates	24 Burney Falls
UTM Zone (WGS 84)	10T
Easting	0613202
Northing	4540833
Latitude	N41° 0.75749′
Longitude	W121° 39.2931′

25 Soda Creek Road to Castle Dome

SCENERY: ✿ ✿ ✿	HIKING TIME: *4 hours*
TRAIL CONDITION: ✿ ✿ ✿ ✿	MAP: *USFS* A Guide to the Mt. Shasta
CHILDREN: ✿ ✿ ✿	Wilderness & Castle Crags Wilderness
DIFFICULTY: ✿	OUTSTANDING FEATURES: *Castle Crags,*
SOLITUDE: ✿	*Indian Springs, Mount Shasta views*
DISTANCE: *8 miles round-trip*	

Standing among the devilish spires of Castle Crags is satiation for the imagination, and the dead-ahead views of Mount Shasta take the breath away, but one of my favorite spots on this hike is magical Indian Springs, halfway to the top.

🚶🚶 To spend some time on the Pacific Crest Trail, access the Crags Trail from the Soda Creek exit on Interstate 5. The PCT winds easily through dense forest for 1.8 miles before linking to the Crags Trail in Castle Crags State Park.

Along the way, a maze of trails crosses the PCT, so be aware. Within the first mile, the historic Kettlebelly Trail comes in from the left, the Root Creek Trail comes in from the right around mile 1.7, and almost immediately after the Vista Trail comes in from the left. Simply continue on the PCT without detouring and you'll be fine.

The junction you want to take is the Crags Trail, which comes up almost immediately after the Vista Trail. Follow the Crags Trail up and stay on the trail until the turnoff to Indian Springs.

Indian Springs is magical because it is such a contrast to the rest of this hike, which is dry through woodlands or exposed on fields of granite. Indian Springs is a lush oasis spewing from a collection of rocks in the middle of the forest. Fresh, clean water (the drinking water for the park) pours out of the mountain and turns everything in its path a verdant green. Fill up your canteens and take the trail back to the Crags Trail.

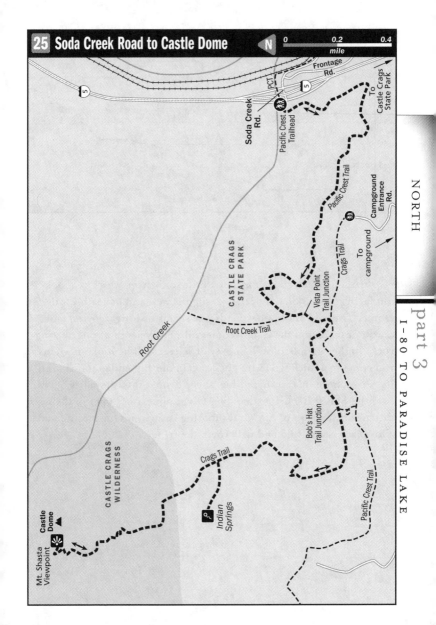

Frontage Rd.

5

PCT

5

To Castle Crags State Park

Soda Creek Rd.

Pacific Crest Trailhead

Pacific Crest Trail

NORTH

Campground Entrance Rd.

To campground

Crags Trail

CASTLE CRAGS STATE PARK

Vista Point Trail Junction

Root Creek Trail

Root Creek

part 3
I-80 TO PARADISE LAKE

Bob's Hat Trail Junction

Crags Trail

Pacific Crest Trail

CASTLE CRAGS WILDERNESS

Indian Springs

Castle Dome

Mt. Shasta Viewpoint

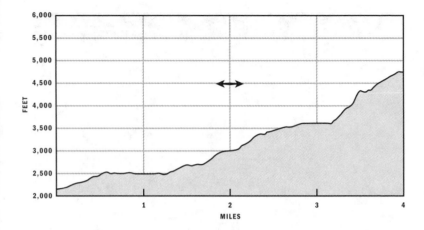

From here it's approximately 1 mile to the top, which is a lookout facing Mount Shasta dead-on, slightly west and beneath Castle Dome. The wild and spooky landscape seems fit for gargoyles, and as you near the top the trail becomes diluted by a web of intersecting rock climber's trails. You'll know you've reached the lookout when you come to a thick steel wire and a steel pole embedded in the granite. From here, it's an incredible, sheer drop-off to the valley below. And the only thing better than Shasta's glimmering slopes in the near distance is the rush of hot wind shooting straight up the granite wall. This place is very wild and well worth the trip.

DIRECTIONS   From Castle Crags State Park, follow I-5 north 0.5 miles to the Soda Creek Road exit. Turn left on Soda Creek Road and follow to its dead end at the green gate.

PERMITS   Wilderness permits are not required for overnight trips into the Castle Crags Wilderness off the Crags Trail. Campfire permits are required and can be obtained in Castle Crags State Park. Camping is available at developed campsites in the state park. Sites are issued on a first-come, first-serve basis, or can be reserved at www.recreation.gov. There is a park entrance fee of $6 per vehicle.

GPS Trailhead Coordinates	25 Soda Creek Road to Castle Dome
UTM Zone (WGS 84)	10T
Easting	0558855
Northing	4557107
Latitude	N41° 09.7895′
Longitude	W122° 17.9075′

NORTH

part 3
I-80 TO PARADISE LAKE

26 Middle Deadfall Lake and Mount Eddy

SCENERY: ✿ ✿ ✿ ✿	Mount Eddy and around Middle Deadfall Lake; 6 miles round-trip to Middle Deadfall Lake
TRAIL CONDITION: ✿ ✿ ✿ ✿ ✿	
CHILDREN: ✿ ✿ ✿ ✿	HIKING TIME: 2–5 hours
DIFFICULTY: ✿	MAP: USFS Shasta-Trinity National Forest
SOLITUDE: ✿ ✿	OUTSTANDING FEATURES: Middle Deadfall Lake, wildflowers, natural spring, views of Mount Shasta from Mount Eddy
DISTANCE: 13.4 miles round-trip to the top of	

There's something for everyone on this easy, hard-packed section of the Pacific Crest Trail; it's a sure crowd pleaser. Ambitious hikers can summit Mount Eddy for extraordinary views of Mount Shasta. For everyone else, there's fishing, swimming, wildflowers, wildlife, and peace and quiet at Middle Deadfall Lake.

🚶 The buzz is out about the hike to Middle Deadfall Lake—it's short, pretty, and lush with wildflowers in midsummer. This hard-packed section of the PCT is flat and fast, perfect for a trail run, with endless views into the Shasta-Trinity National Forest, Trinity River basin, and lush Deadfall Meadow below.

Along the PCT you come to a hillside spring spilling over the trail with a vibrant swath of Indian paintbrush blooming in its path. Shortly after the spring, the trail crosses Deadfall Creek and you reach a spaghetti bowl of trails. The PCT heads right (south) to Deadfall Meadow and Toad Lake, while the Mount Eddy Trail and Sisson Callahan Trail continue to Middle Deadfall Lake (straight ahead).

At the next fork in the trail, bear right to reach Middle Deadfall Lake just over the rise. Bearing left you continue to steadily climb up past Middle Deadfall Lake toward Mount Eddy.

Spending the day at Middle Deadfall Lake, the largest of the three Deadfall Lakes, is relaxing. You can lounge on the rocks around the

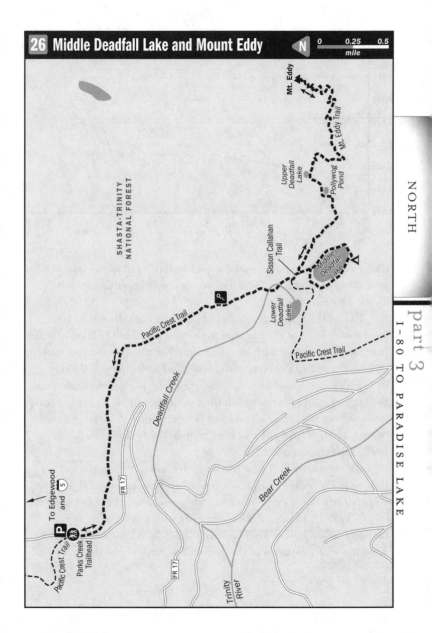

Mt. Eddy

Mt. Eddy Trail

Upper
Deadfall
Lake

Pollywog
Pond

SHASTA-TRINITY
NATIONAL FOREST

NORTH

Sisson Callahan
Trail

Middle
Deadfall
Lake

Pacific Crest Trail

Lower
Deadfall
Lake

Pacific Crest Trail

part 3
I–80 TO PARADISE LAKE

Deadfall Creek

To Edgewood
and (5)

FR 17

Bear Creek

Pacific Crest Trail

P

Parks Creek
Trailhead

FR 17

Trinity
River

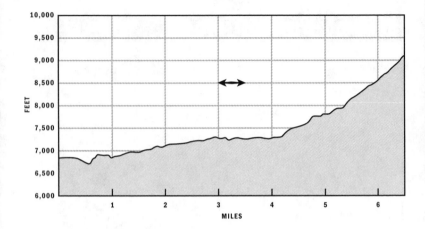

lake, camp, fish, or swim, and there's a trail that circles the lake so it's possible to create space if you find yourself wanting your own sub-alpine-lake paradise.

Two of the biggest campsites are at opposite sides of the lake, lengthwise. Most of the bugs are at the south end of the lake. On the northeast end, a patch of interesting pitcher plants is worth a look.

After circling the lake, swimming, and lounging you'll likely be eager to check out the top of Mount Eddy. It's a nice climb, and although it might look intimidating, the trail follows a pretty consis-tent grade to the top. To reach the summit, trace the trail you took to Middle Deadfall Lake and keep right at the fork. From there it's pretty self-explanatory.

On the way, you'll pass two water features. At first glance, the first one, Pollywog Pond, looks much less than spectacular—a green, stagnant, shallow pond. At second glance, during the third week of July anyway, I realized it was teeming with a million or more tadpoles—what a great place to bring the kids! There's one nice campsite at the east end of the pond. The trail circles the pond and

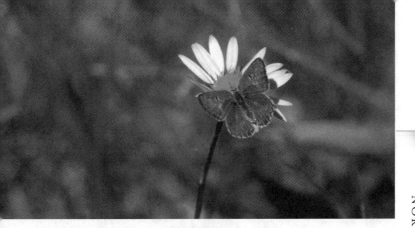

California aster is one of the many kinds of wildflowers on this hike.

shortly passes another lake. The second feature is Upper Deadfall Lake and is suitable, although not desirable, for swimming. There's also a nice campsite here on the east end of the lake, under the shadow of Mount Eddy.

To reach the summit of Mount Eddy, pass the lake and start the real climb to its shoulder. Here the Sisson Callahan Trail continues east to the North Fork of the Sacramento River and the Mount Eddy Trail heads left and switchbacks right up to the summit. There's an incredible selection of wildflowers up here, even for the dry climate (in season, of course).

At the top of Mount Eddy (9,025 feet) you'll find a reward in the shape of Mount Shasta staring you right in the face. Mount Eddy is the northernmost point of the Shasta-Trinity Divide; snowmelt from its east flank flows into the Sacramento River, off its north flank flows into the Klamath River, and from its west flank empties into the Trinity River. This summit was also a fire lookout at one time as evidenced by the stacks of abandoned lumber at the summit.

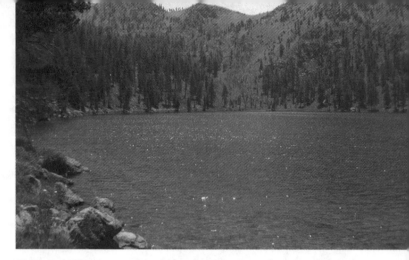

Middle Deadfall Lake, named for the trees that fall into it, is (at 25 acres) the largest of the three Deadfall Lakes.

DIRECTIONS   From Interstate 5 north of Weed, take the Edgewood exit and drive northwest on old Highway 99 for 0.5 miles. Turn left on Stewart Springs Road and drive to the road's end. Turn right on FS 17 and drive 10 miles to the Deadfall Lakes (Parks Creek) parking area.

GPS Trailhead Coordinates	26 Middle Deadfall Lake and Mount Eddy
UTM Zone (WGS 84)	10T
Easting	0538668
Northing	4576930
Latitude	N41° 20.5761'
Longitude	W122° 32.2694'

27 Statue Lake

SCENERY: ✿ ✿ ✿ ✿	DISTANCE: *7 miles round-trip*
TRAIL CONDITION: ✿ ✿ ✿	HIKING TIME: *1–2 hours*
CHILDREN: ✿ ✿ ✿ ✿ ✿	MAP: *USFS* A Guide to the Marble Mountain Wilderness & Russian Wilderness
DIFFICULTY: ✿ ✿	
SOLITUDE: ✿ ✿ ✿ ✿	OUTSTANDING FEATURES: *Statue Lake, great day hike for artists*

Statue Lake's tucked-away location makes finding this natural artistic wonder like finding the Holy Grail. Within an hour you'll be pondering the goddess of granite's sculpture.

🏃 This hike starts off much like the hike to Paynes Lake or the Big Blue Lake (see Hike 29, page 159). Start at the Music Creek Trailhead and follow the well-worn switchbacks through pine forest about a mile up to the intersection with the Pacific Crest Trail. Take a right and travel south on the PCT. From here, it's a nice walk over a mostly flat, consistent gradient exactly 1.2 miles to a creek crossing.

You may notice an established campsite on the right of the PCT and a faint trail starting up the creek bed to the left. Statue Lake lies sunken in a ring of guardian granite boulders, and if you follow this creek up the hill you will find the lake.

Beware, there isn't a trail, but the forest is not so thick and it's easy to follow the gradient of the slope. You'll know you're getting close to the lake when you start seeing more granite boulders littering the slope. Follow these boulders, like bread crumbs, to hidden Statue Lake.

Another route, although not as direct, continues on the PCT to a sharp bend in the trail. A ridge scattered with big granite boulders rises to your left at your first hairpin turn on the PCT, approximately 200 yards after the creek. Forge off-trail, again, following the boulders like bread crumbs along the ridgeline to Statue Lake. It's

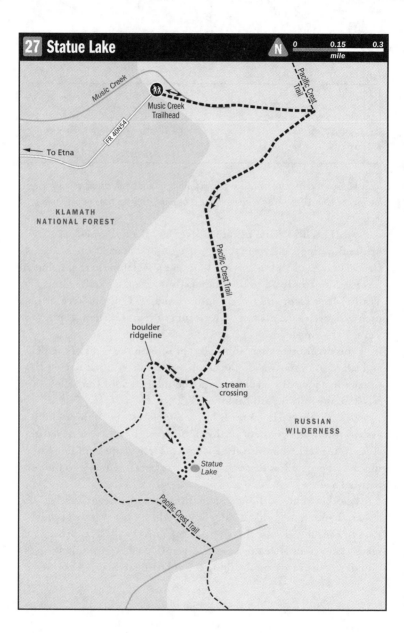

N

0   0.15   0.3
mile

Music Creek

Music Creek
Trailhead

FR 40N54

← To Etna

Pacific Crest
Trail

KLAMATH
NATIONAL FOREST

Pacific Crest Trail

boulder
ridgeline

stream
crossing

RUSSIAN
WILDERNESS

Statue
Lake

Pacific Crest Trail

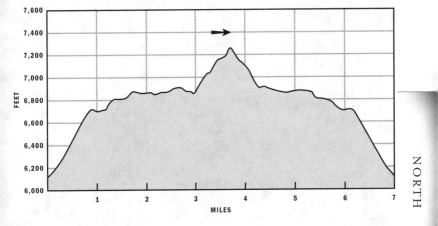

approximately 0.5 miles from the PCT. Following the stream, it's approximately 0.3 miles.

Once you get to Statue Lake, there's not much to do except stare at the incredible natural artwork of the lake and its granite fortress. It doesn't take much to imagine a goddess of granite artwork chiseling the sharp, jagged outline of the lake's south side. Two distinct statuelike figures tower above the lake as stone soldiers looking out into the vast Russian Wilderness beyond.

There are many boulders piled around the lake, but not many are completely flat. One nice flat spot could make a great campsite for two people maximum or one person comfortably. This place would be great for an outdoor painter to set up a canvas and attempt to capture this natural inspiration.

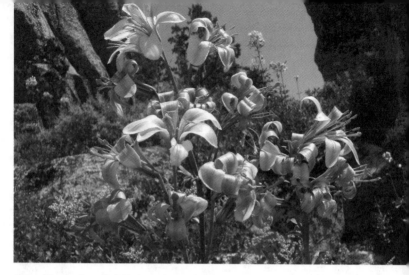

Sierra lilies brighten the hillside just beyond the granite sculptures framing the east side of Statue Lake.

DIRECTIONS   From Interstate 5 at Yreka, take the CA 3/Fort Jones exit and drive 28 miles southwest to Etna. Turn west on Etna–Somes Bar Road and drive 20 miles. Just before the Salmon River Bridge, turn left on FS 40N54 and drive 10 miles to the Music Creek Trailhead. (This drive takes a little longer than an hour from Etna.)

PERMITS   No permits are required for the Russian Wilderness Area, but groups are limited to 25 persons.

GPS Trailhead Coordinates	27 Statue Lake
UTM Zone (WGS 84)	10T
Easting	0502755
Northing	4575533
Latitude	N41° 19.8761′
Longitude	W122° 58.0246′

SCENERY: ✿ ✿ ✿ ✿ ✿	*Big Blue Lake, 12.7 miles round-trip*
TRAIL CONDITION: ✿ ✿	HIKING TIME: *2–6 hours*
CHILDREN: ✿ ✿ ✿	MAP: *USFS* A Guide to the Marble Mountain Wilderness & Russian Wilderness
DIFFICULTY: ✿ ✿ ✿ ✿	
SOLITUDE: ✿ ✿ ✿ ✿	OUTSTANDING FEATURES: *Paynes Lake, Upper Albert Lake, Big Blue Lake, exciting route-finding*
DISTANCE: *Paynes Lake, 5 miles round-trip;*	

The only folks you will see out here are the ones who know this land intimately. Once people find this nook of backcountry nirvana, they return time and time again. While Paynes Lake is a family day hike or overnighter with great fishing, the Big Blue Lake Loop beckons adventurers who like to travel off-trail to see wild and scenic places.

🥾 From the Music Creek Trailhead, the trail gradually climbs a series of long switchbacks through thick forest for about 1 mile to an intersection with the Pacific Crest Trail. Paynes Lake is about another mile north of this intersection.

At the junction, head left (north) as the trail climbs gradually through the remaining forest. After about 0.5 miles, the character of the trail changes dramatically and all of the sudden you're hugging a bare, granite-bouldered ridgeline with a clear view of the Russian Wilderness.

As you gradually descend to the turnoff to Paynes Lake, you pass Lipstick Lake, a murky pond hundreds of feet below the trail. At the first substantial creek crossing, you come to an intersection with the Paynes Lake Trail. To head up to the lake, take a left.

Paynes Lake is a warm lake with a soggy, mucky bottom that's great for fishing (anglers will find eastern brook and rainbow trout) but not for swimming because the area's used to graze cattle. This lake is also popular with backcountry equestrians. There's great camping at Paynes Lake; the wooded shoreline feels parklike.

For an adventure in alpine lake hunting, follow the north side of Paynes Lake to a marshy area where a small creek cascades the slope

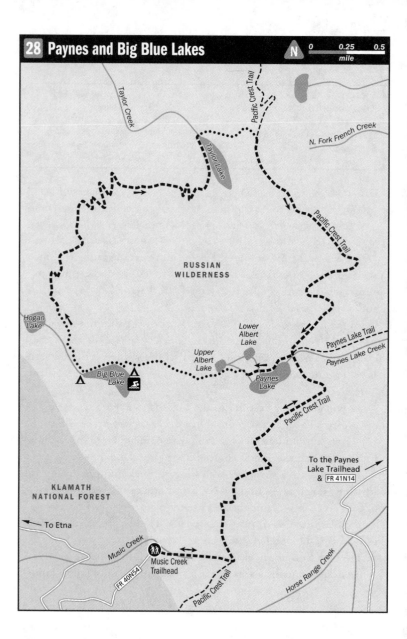

N

0   0.25   0.5
mile

Taylor Creek

Pacific Crest Trail

Taylor Lake

N. Fork French Creek

Pacific Crest Trail

RUSSIAN
WILDERNESS

Hogan
Lake

Lower
Albert
Lake

Paynes Lake Trail

Upper
Albert
Lake

Paynes Lake Creek

Big Blue
Lake

Paynes
Lake

Pacific Crest Trail

To the Paynes
Lake Trailhead
& FR 41N14

KLAMATH
NATIONAL FOREST

To Etna

Music Creek

Music Creek
Trailhead

FR 40N54

Pacific Crest Trail

Horse Range Creek

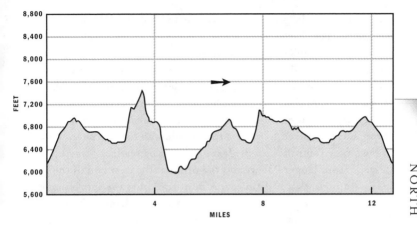

at the back of the lake. From here, start your journey off-trail. The easiest way up the slope is to follow the large talus field just left of the steep, grassy creek bed. Aim for what looks like a low spot or saddle in the mountain.

The climb goes rather quickly to Lower Albert Lake, another mucky, shallow lake. From here, follow a faint trail left around the bottom of the lake toward a creek that pours into Lower Albert Lake. Then follow this creek up to Upper Albert Lake, great for swimming and set in a ring of granite.

Upper Albert Lake is a worthy day-hike destination and a great out-of-the-way spot to take in the serenity and just relax. But for the ultimate day hike, read on—there are still more lakes to see.

From Upper Albert Lake, stay right, climbing the blocky, granite slope. When I scouted this hike, I nicknamed this patch of non-trail "bumblebee pass" because in late July the fuzzy bees swarm the ubiquitous pink and purple tufts of wildflowers dispersed between chalky, granite boulders. They're relatively harmless, but they're everywhere.

Aim for the saddle of this slope and soon you find yourself overlooking Big Blue Lake, an enormous, secluded lake with a nice, granite bottom. It's so clear and cool that it was probably the best swimming lake I hiked to all season—and that's saying a lot!

From the saddle, it's a very steep scree field descent to Big Blue. There's a faint trail at first, but you'll eventually need to find your own way. It is an excruciatingly difficult descent and can take almost an hour to complete. The swim, however, is worth it.

I can't imagine carrying a fully loaded backpack down this slope, but I've talked to quite a few people who have done it. There are two nice campsites on the lake: one just beneath the steep descent from Upper Albert and the other at the west end of the lake, although it's a little buggy. A faint trail hugs the shoreline on the west end of the lake, where a small trickle of water leaks out of Big Blue and tumbles down a shallow cleft in the granite slope leading to Hogan Lake.

To complete this loop, continue off-trail to Hogan Lake. It takes quite a leap of faith, but stay slightly right of the trickle and look out for the odd cairn here and there.

After the descent, the route doesn't pass directly by Hogan Lake, but anglers looking for eastern brook and rainbow trout might like to detour. Hogan Meadow is outstanding, but is also used for cattle grazing, so the trail through the meadow can be difficult to follow. The trail leaving the meadow is not very scenic and climbs moderately to an overlook of Taylor Lake.

From here, your route to the trailhead is right in front of your eyes, but when you first see it you may think it impossible. The task is to follow the trail to Taylor Lake and around the bottom of the lake, where the stream empties out (which is to stay left). From here, swing around the bottom and up the opposite side of the lake via a chunky, talus field. From the top, it looks impossible, but it's possible. Aim for the saddle again, and you'll be pleasantly surprised to find the well-traveled, neatly marked PCT.

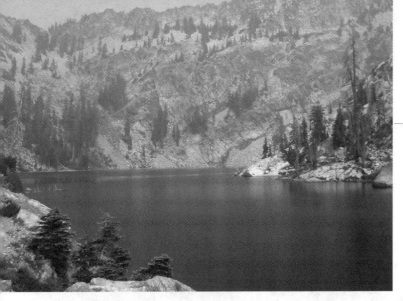

All you'll find at secluded Big Blue Lake in the Russian Wilderness is excellent swimming and stunning views.

Head right (south) on the PCT to connect with the Music Creek Trailhead past Paynes Lake, and that's your lollipop ultra-route-finding day hike. While this loop is not for beginner hikers, it's a great adventure if you're well prepared.

After hiking, make sure to stop by the Etna Brewery, in business since 1872, just off main street in downtown Etna. Enjoy the fine dark-beer selection and the Blackberry Blonde Ale.

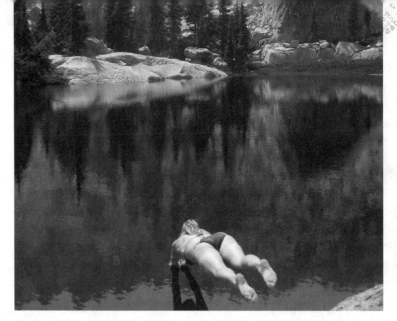

A dip in refreshing Upper Albert Lake is a great way to break up this arduous hike.

DIRECTIONS   From Interstate 5 at Yreka, take the CA 3/Fort Jones exit and drive 28 miles southwest to Etna. Turn west on Etna–Somes Bar Road and drive 20 miles. Just before the Salmon River Bridge, turn left on FS 40N54 and drive 10 miles to the Music Creek Trailhead. (This drive takes a little longer than an hour from Etna.)

PERMITS   No permits are required for the Russian Wilderness Area, but groups are limited to 25 persons.

GPS Trailhead Coordinates	28 Paynes and Big Blue Lakes
UTM Zone (WGS 84)	10T
Easting	0502755
Northing	4575533
Latitude	N41° 19.8761′
Longitude	W122° 58.0246′

29 Little Elk Lake

SCENERY: ⛺ ⛺ ⛺	DISTANCE: *19.7 miles*
TRAIL CONDITION: ⛺ ⛺	HIKING TIME: *10 hours or 2 days*
CHILDREN: ⛺	MAP: *USFS* A Guide to the Marble Mountain Wilderness & Russian Wilderness
DIFFICULTY: ⛺ ⛺ ⛺ ⛺ ⛺	
SOLITUDE: ⛺ ⛺ ⛺ ⛺	OUTSTANDING FEATURES: *Lake views, natural springs, route-finding*

Competent hikers without fear of the wild moo-cow and with a penchant for circumnavigating behemoth, unnamed mountain peaks need only apply for this near 20-mile challenge in the Marble Mountain Wilderness.

🚶🚶 A good way to get an early start on this grueling day hike is to pitch a tent at the Shackleford Trailhead, which has a few nice campsites, a small parking area, an outhouse, and a large corral that often hosts herds of horses. The trail climbs steadily just out of view of the noisy Shackleford Creek through the Marble Mountain Wilderness. Along the way, a handful of natural springs seep from the hillside and over the trail.

After mid-July, quite a few cattle make this area their summer grazing grounds. At just less than 1 mile along the trail, watch where you walk; you're sharing the trail with cow patties! That's not to say the trail isn't scenic. It meanders through a pretty mix of conifers, deciduous trees, and nice meadows. And overall, it's much less dusty than a lot of the other trails in the area.

Keep right (north) at the first junction to Log Lake and Campbell Lake. Shortly afterward, Log Lake, a shallow pond overgrown with lily pads, comes into sight on your left. Stay left (west) at the turnoff to Calf Lake, and within another mile veer right (west) toward Summit Lake. Soon you begin to see signs of a change in the landscape. While densely forested hillsides dominated the landscape previously, marbled boulders now pave an

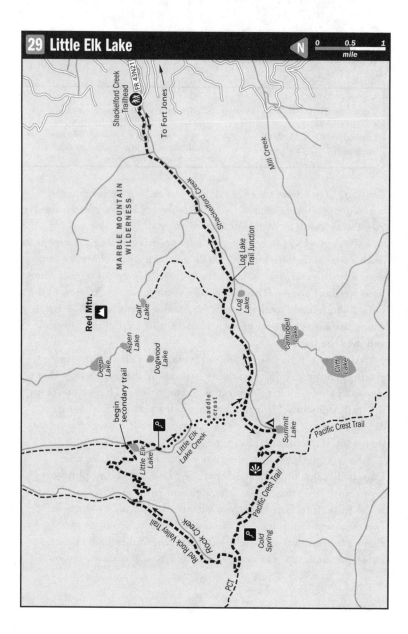

N

0   0.5   1
mile

Shackelford Creek Trailhead

FR 43N21

To Fort Jones

MARBLE MOUNTAIN WILDERNESS

Shackelford Creek

Mill Creek

Log Lake Trail Junction

Calf Lake

Log Lake

Campbell Lake

Red Mtn.

Aspen Lake

Dogwood Lake

Cliff Lake

Deep Lake

begin secondary trail

saddle crest

Little Elk Lake Creek

Little Elk Lake

Summit Lake

Pacific Crest Trail

Pacific Crest Trail

Red Rock Valley Trail

Rock Creek

Cold Spring

PCT

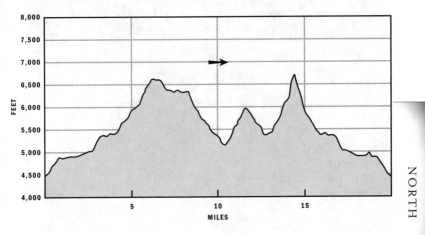

irregular path to the top of the steep slope to the north (your right) of the trail.

Pay particular attention to this area—it is in the vicinity of the return trip from Little Elk Lake. The return route follows a secondary trail (cross-country route), which is often obscured by stray game and cattle trails. Within a mile of the boulder field you reach Summit Lake, a nice lake for fishing, with a few good spots for swimming and a popular campsite with hikers (and not so much with equestrians). I advise overnighters to drop their bulky gear here before completing the rest of this aggressive loop-hike, but make sure to bring a water filter and your map for the remaining portion of the loop.

The ascent picks up a notch or two after Summit Lake and doesn't let up until reaching a scenic overlook approximately 0.5 miles later. From the overlook, there are impressive views of Summit Lake below, Campbell Lake farther in the distance, and the steep bowl south of Summit Lake that hides Cliff Lake.

About 200 yards past the stunning overlook (which makes a nice snack spot) is the intersection with the Pacific Crest Trail. Turn right

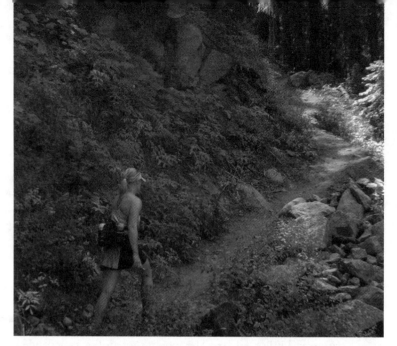

Shortly after crossing Rock Creek, the trail to Little Elk Lake climbs through shady forest.

at the intersection and continue northwest on the PCT. The views from the sunny ridgeline into Big Elk Fork and Wooley Creek canyons to the west are stunning. This side of the ridge is overgrown with wildflowers in early to midsummer, and the few times the trail ducks into cool, shady mountain hemlock forest is a cool respite from the heat common later in the summer months.

After 2 miles of relatively easy walking on the PCT, turn right to drop into Red Rock Valley (heading more northeast) inhabited by friendly cows.

Follow the main trail through the canyon for exactly 2 miles past the turnoff. A few times throughout the valley, cow paths cross the main trail and head off into various directions; the trail to Little Elk Lake is clearly marked by a prominent intersection and a sign.

Immediately after making the right turn east to Little Elk, you cross Rock Creek. The trail begins following the creek upstream to start and goes past some decent pools for filtering water. By this time your canteen is probably running close to dry, and this is the last place to fill up before a relatively steep climb and descent to Little Elk Lake. Be aware that you probably won't feel like filling up at Little Elk because the lake is overrun with cattle.

On the way to Little Elk, you'll climb approximately 900 feet in the first mile and will then descend another 600 feet over the next 1.4 miles of switchbacks before reaching the lake. Follow the trail to the outflow of the lake; directly across the stream there is an unmarked fork. The well-traveled path heads left (north), gradually ascending to Deep Lake; the less-traveled path heads right (south) and around Little Elk Lake.

This is where the adventure begins. Follow the less-traveled path south and be prepared for some route-finding. Climb along the small drainage at the south (or far) end of the lake after leaving lake level as the sound of running water gets louder and louder.

Follow the noise of the water to a spring gushing out of the mountainside and tumbling over enormous boulders. It is heaven on earth. After leaving Little Elk Lake thirsty, the idea of fresh, clean water is electrifying.

Fill up here because the climb continues as you complete the circumnavigation of the enormous unnamed peak, a textbook example of glacial terrain, now to your right. You may find cairns loosely marking the faint, unmaintained trail all the way up to another meadow and marshy area.

From this meadow, you climb 600 feet in less than 0.25 miles. It's steep, and the trail is faint in places. It can be difficult to find the correct route. From the marshy meadow, hang right (west) around the low spot. Contour around the west side of the meadow until you find a faint trail that climbs up through the middle forested swath of the bowl and heads directly for the westernmost saddle on the ridge.

Cresting this ridge brings an incredible feeling of accomplishment, and you're rewarded with fantastic views of Little Elk Lake, Campbell Lake, Summit Lake, and miles and miles of river canyons. The trail down from the saddle is also hard to follow, but it mainly heads downhill and to the left (east) before connecting with the Shackleford Creek Trail. There are no impassable cliffs, but the trail is slick and dusty in places. Just be prepared. It's reassuring (in a way) to see evidence that our four-legged friends (the moo-cows) have made it up this far. If they can do it, so can you.

DIRECTIONS   From Interstate 5 at Yreka, take the CA 3/Fort Jones exit. Drive 16.5 miles to Fort Jones and turn right on Scott River Road. Follow Scott River Road 7 miles before turning left on Quartz Valley Road. Drive 4 miles to the sign for Shackleford Creek. Turn right onto Forest Road 43N21; continue 7 miles to the end of the road where you'll find the trailhead.

PERMITS   No permits are required for ovenight stays in the Marble Mountain Wilderness.

GPS Trailhead Coordinates	29 Little Elk Lake
UTM Zone (WGS 84)	10T
Easting	0495904
Northing	4601214
Latitude	N41° 33.7553′
Longitude	W123° 2.9474′

30 Shadow Lake

SCENERY: ☆ ☆ ☆ ☆
TRAIL CONDITION: ☆ ☆ ☆ ☆
CHILDREN: ☆ ☆ ☆ ☆
DIFFICULTY: ☆ ☆ ☆
SOLITUDE: ☆ ☆ ☆ ☆ ☆

DISTANCE: *15.2 miles round-trip*
HIKING TIME: *6–8 hours or 2 days*
MAP: *USFS* A Guide to the Marble Mountain Wilderness & Russian Wilderness
OUTSTANDING FEATURES: *Shadow Lake, views of the Marble Mountains, marble valleys*

Imagine your own natural pool overlooking deep river canyons and the Marble Mountains—bleached white, red, and black mounds of rugged rock. That's Shadow Lake. Locals begged me not to write about it, but you'll be happy I did.

🏃 There couldn't be a more idyllic starting point for the overnight destination of Shadow Lake than Lovers Camp Trailhead. It's just a simple, no-fee parking lot with a few sites, a couple of picnic tables, and a troubled bear here and there, but it's lovely. However, there is no potable water available; the horse camp, just 0.25 miles down the road, has a running faucet.

The trail following Canyon Creek extends deep into the Marble Mountain Wilderness all the way to the backbone of the Pacific Crest Trail 4.4 miles from the start. Along the way, you travel through shady, deciduous forest. Berry bushes—blackberries, wild strawberries, chokeberries, and wild blueberries—and mushrooms are interspersed along the way. It is a great place to bring the field guide, and a favorite trail among foragers—take the bears, for instance. Note that bear canisters are not required in this area and are not even available at local ranger stations. For your safety, minimize the amount of fragrant substances in your vehicle before hiking.

The trail climbs gradually through the thick forest populated by incense cedars, mountain hemlocks, firs, and a mix of other trees. Along the way you'll see three forks: the first, within a mile of the

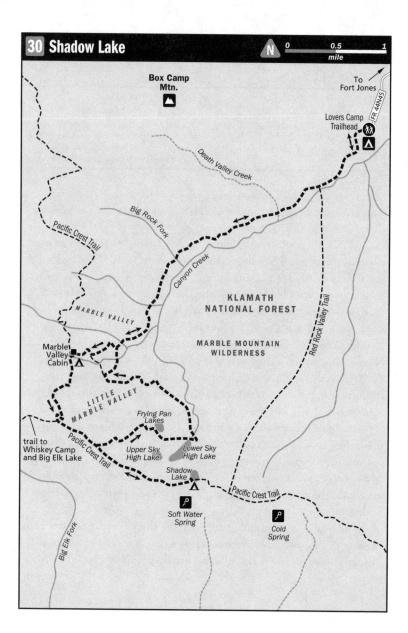

N

0   0.5   1
mile

Box Camp
Mtn.

To
Fort Jones

Lovers Camp
Trailhead

FR 44N45

Death Valley Creek

Big Rock Fork

Pacific Crest Trail

Canyon Creek

KLAMATH
NATIONAL
FOREST

MARBLE VALLEY

MARBLE MOUNTAIN
WILDERNESS

Red Rock Valley Trail

Marble
Valley
Cabin

LITTLE
MARBLE VALLEY

Frying Pan
Lakes

trail to
Whiskey Camp
and Big Elk Lake

Pacific Crest Trail

Upper Sky
High Lake

Lower Sky
High Lake

Shadow
Lake

Pacific Crest Trail

Soft Water
Spring

Cold
Spring

Big Elk Fork

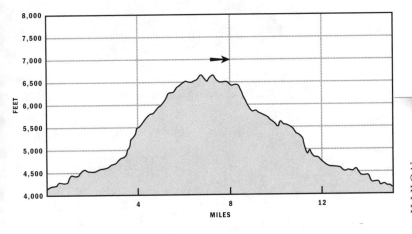

start, to Red Rock Valley and the remaining two to Marble Valley and Marble Valley Cabin. Keep right every time.

After approximately 4 miles of hiking, you begin to see ribbons of marble veins in the hillside. This marble, which was once limestone, still exhibits the cavernous qualities of the stone, and there are plenty of small caves off the trail. Just before you reach the intersection with the PCT, there's an incredible view of the Marble Mountains, strikingly white towering above the meadow, at Marble Valley Cabin. This cabin, built in the 1920s by the U.S. Forest Service as a fire detector camp, is used only for Forest Service administration and is, unfortunately, not open to the public.

Travel south on the PCT through an area covered with lush wildflowers early to midsummer. In about 2 miles you reach an unmarked turn to the left, which is the route to Shadow Lake.

Before this unmarked fork, after 1 mile of walking along the ridge, you pass the marked intersection to Big Elk Lake and Whiskey Camp. The first turnoff to Sky High Lakes is about 0.5 miles farther. The next turnoff is the most direct route to Shadow Lake.

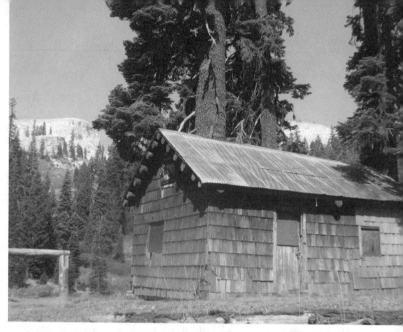

Marble Valley Cabin, administered by the U.S. Forest Service, is not open to the public. But the incredible views of the Marble Mountain are free for everyone to enjoy.

Shadow Lake is exactly 0.5 miles away from the PCT. The faint trail passes through fields of California asters and stands of mountain hemlock. While not ideal for swimming, Shadow Lake is fantastic for wildlife watching and stocked with eastern brook trout. Newts rise and sink slowly from the lake's surface to its seaweed-blanketed bottom. There's only one nice swimming spot. It is small but is located right at the campsite looking out at the Marble Mountains. The site is also a stone's throw away from a dramatic view of the Sky High Lakes below.

Perched on this out-of-the-way wooded bench, Shadow is a quiet retreat and a world of its own. Falling asleep under the stars and watching morning's first rosy light splash across Black Marble Mountain is an unforgettable sight.

For the return trip you have a choice: You can add a mile by making the lake loop past Frying Pan and the Sky High lakes, or you can make the trip an out-and-back by following the PCT back to Marble Valley Cabin. Admittedly, Sky High Lakes are not too special, although they do have a lot of fish. This area is also popular with backcountry equestrians. In fact, I was once confronted with a runaway horse whose owner I never met!

DIRECTIONS   From Interstate 5 at Yreka take the CA 3/Fort Jones exit. Drive 16.5 miles to Fort Jones and turn right on Scott River Road; follow it 14 miles. Turn left at Indian Scotty Campground Road and go 1 mile. Keep slightly left at Forest Route 44N45 and follow it 5.3 miles. Turn left onto Forest Route 43N45. Continue on FR 43N45 approximately 1.5 miles before reaching Lovers Camp Trailhead.

PERMITS   No permits are required for overnight stays in Marble Mountain Wilderness.

GPS Trailhead Coordinates	30 Shadow Lake
UTM Zone (WGS 84)	10T
Easting	0488136
Northing	4604767
Latitude	N41° 35.6711'
Longitude	W123° 8.5416'

31 Paradise Lake

SCENERY: ✿ ✿	HIKING TIME: *4–6 hours*
TRAIL CONDITION: ✿ ✿ ✿	MAP: *USFS* A Guide to the Marble Mountain Wilderness & Russian Wilderness
CHILDREN: ✿ ✿ ✿	
DIFFICULTY: ✿ ✿ ✿	OUTSTANDING FEATURES: *Fishing in Paradise and Bear lakes, historic trails, lush wildflowers in early summer*
SOLITUDE: ✿ ✿ ✿	
DISTANCE: *8 miles*	

Ascend to one of the Marble Mountains' most accessible lakes and relish the opportunity to hike two historic trails—the PCT and Kelsey Creek Trail—while enjoying lush wildflowers in early summer.

🚶🚶 At the Paradise Lake Trailhead, a sign and map bear the words, "Retreat from civilization, reconnect with the Earth, and find healing, meaning, and significance . . . In contrast with areas where man and his works dominate the landscape, hereby is recognized as an area where the Earth is a community of life untrammeled by man." It's the entrance to 227,000 acres of land in the Marble Mountain Wilderness, which is protected from resource extraction, roads, and development. However, the statement "untrammeled by man" is a little far-fetched. This densely forested and rugged area is also heavily frequented by ranchers whose cattle spend the summers grazing the subalpine meadows.

The 2-mile ascent to Paradise Lake is a steep series of dusty switchbacks through thick mixed conifer forest. Near the top of the grade, a colorful hillside comes into view before you reach Paradise Lake. After 2 miles of walking along the Paradise Creek Trail, turn right at the junction with the PCT, and shortly after the intersection Paradise Lake comes into view.

Paradise Lake is a shallow lake, not terribly well suited for swimming and alright for fishing. It's a popular campsite for equestrians, and for hunters beginning in September, when elk season opens.

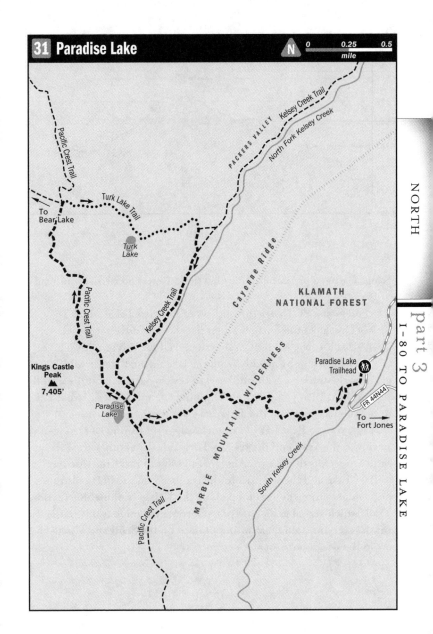

31 Paradise Lake

N 0   0.25   0.5
         mile

NORTH

part 3
I-80 TO PARADISE LAKE

Pacific Crest Trail

Kelsey Creek Trail

PACKERS VALLEY

North Fork Kelsey Creek

To Bear Lake

Turk Lake Trail

Turk Lake

Pacific Crest Trail

Kelsey Creek Trail

Cayenne Ridge

KLAMATH
NATIONAL FOREST

Kings Castle Peak
▲
7,405'

Paradise Lake

MARBLE MOUNTAIN WILDERNESS

Pacific Crest Trail

Paradise Lake
Trailhead

FR 44N44

To
Fort Jones

South Kelsey Creek

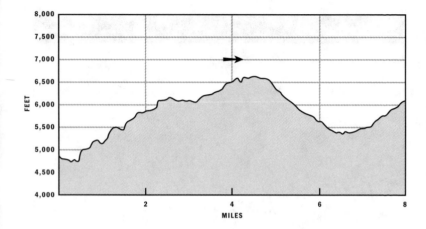

Kings Castle, a prominent marbled peak, towers above the south side of Paradise Lake.

Follow the PCT over the outflow of Paradise Lake, which is Kelsey Creek. At the outflow a sign points toward Kelsey Creek Trail—this historic route is your return trail for this semiloop hike.

The PCT climbs steadily from the lake through dense wildflowers in early summer. Vibrant fireweed towers overhead on the uphill side of the trail as you continue climbing 1.5 miles past Paradise Lake to the intersection with the Turk Lake and Bear Lake trails.

The trail to Bear Lake (a notoriously good fishing lake) descends steeply to the west, and the trail to Turk Lake (overrun with grazing cattle) descends to the east. Anglers will want to make the side trip to Bear Lake and then return to the trailhead on the PCT. History buffs might enjoy the semiloop along the Kelsey National Recreation Trail, which served as a primary trade route for mule trains in the 1850s, carrying gold from mining camps on the Scott and Shasta rivers to the ocean ports near Crescent City.

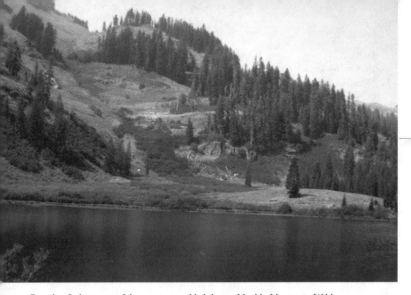

Paradise Lake is one of the most accessible lakes in Marble Mountain Wilderness.

To access Kelsey Trail, descend toward Turk Lake on a rough, steep, and rocky trail to the small lake. You'll most likely hear a cacophony of cowbells. The trail vanishes here and there but mostly heads downhill and left (northeast) of Turk Lake.

At the northeast corner of Turk Lake, at the edge of a pine forest, there is a fire pit. Exactly to the left of the fire pit, the trail descends to Kelsey Creek through thick tree cover. From Turk Lake it's approximately 0.5 miles to the Kelsey Creek Trail; bear right at the intersection. Kelsey Creek rambles noisily over steep, narrow drops well away from the trail as it climbs up to Paradise Lake through thick wildflower fields and underneath towering cottonwoods.

DIRECTIONS   From Interstate 5, exit at Yreka and follow CA 3 for 16.5 miles into Fort Jones. Turn right on Scott River Road and drive 18 miles before making a left onto the turnoff for Indian Scotty Campground. Continue 6 miles on FS 44N44, then follow signs to the Paradise Lake Trailhead, which is at the end of FS 44N44.

GPS Trailhead Coordinates   31 Paradise Lake
UTM Zone (WGS 84)   10T
Northing   0484777
Easting   4607192
Latitude   N41° 36.9778'
Longitude   W123° 10.9630'

Appendix A: Park Contacts

CASTLE CRAGS STATE PARK
www.parks.ca.gov/default.
  asp?page_id=454
P.O. Box 80
Castella, CA 96017
(530) 235-2684

DEVILS POSTPILE NATIONAL MONUMENT
www.nps.gov/depo
P.O. Box 3999
Mammoth Lakes, CA 93546
(760) 934-2289

ELDORADO NATIONAL FOREST
www.fs.fed.us/r5/eldorado
100 Forni Road
Placerville, CA 95667
(530) 622-5061
TTY: (530) 642-5122

HUMBOLDT-TOIYABE NATIONAL FOREST
www.fs.fed.us/r4/htnf
1200 Franklin Way
Sparks, NV 89431
(775) 331-6444

Bridgeport Ranger District
HC 62, Box 1000
Bridgeport, CA 93517
(760) 932-7070

INYO NATIONAL FOREST
www.fs.fed.us/r5/inyo/about
Mammoth Lakes Visitor Center
2520 Main Street
Mammoth Lakes, CA 93546

Info/Shuttle: (760) 924-5500
Permits: (760) 873-2483

KLAMATH NATIONAL FOREST
www.fs.fed.us/r5/klamath
1312 Fairlane Road
Yreka, CA 96097

Happy Camp/Oak Knoll Ranger District
63822 Highway 96
P.O. Box 377
Happy Camp, CA 96039
(530) 493-2243
TDD: (530) 493-1777

Salmon/Scott River Ranger Districts
11263 N. Highway 3
Fort Jones, CA 96032
(530) 468-5351
TDD: (530) 468-1298

LAKE TAHOE BASIN MANAGEMENT UNIT
www.fs.fed.us/r5/ltbmu
U.S. Forest Service
35 College Drive
South Lake Tahoe, CA 96150
(530) 543-2600
TTY-TDD: (530) 543-0956

LASSEN VOLCANIC NATIONAL PARK
www.nps.gov/lavo
P.O. Box 100
Mineral, CA 96063
(530) 595-4480

McArthur-Burney Memorial Falls State Park

www.parks.ca.gov/?page_id=455
24898 Highway 89
Burney, CA 96013
(530) 335-2777

Pacific Crest Trail Association

www.pcta.org
1331 Garden Highway
Sacramento, CA 95833
(916) 285-1846

Shasta-Trinity National Forest

www.fs.fed.us/r5/shastatrinity

USDA Service Center
Shasta-Trinity National Forest
3644 Avtech Parkway
Redding, CA 96002
(530) 226-2500
TTY-TDD: (530) 226-2490

McCloud Ranger Station
P.O. Box 1620
2019 Forest Road
McCloud, CA 96057
(530) 964-2184
TTY-TDD: (530) 964-2692

Mount Shasta Ranger Station
204 West Alma
Mt. Shasta, CA 96067
(530) 926-4511

Stanislaus National Forest

www.fs.fed.us/r5/stanislaus

Amador Ranger District
26820 Silver Drive
Pioneer, CA 95666
(209) 295-4251

Calaveras Ranger District
5519 Highway 4, P.O. Box 500
Hathaway Pines, CA 95233
(209) 795-1381

Summit Ranger District
#1 Pinecrest Lake Road
Pinecrest, CA 95364
(209) 965-3434
TDD: (209) 965-0488

Tahoe National Forest

www.fs.fed.us/r5/tahoe

Truckee Ranger District
9646 Donner Pass Road
Truckee CA 96161
(530) 587-3558
TDD: (530) 587-6907

Yuba River Ranger District
15924 Highway 49
Camptonville, CA 95922
(530) 288-3231 or 478-6253
TDD: (530) 288-3656
TTY-TDD: (530) 926-4512

Yosemite National Park

www.nps.gov/yose
P.O. Box 577
Yosemite, CA 95389

Tuolumne Meadows Ranger Station
(209) 372-0309

Wilderness Permit Reservations
(209) 372-0740

Visitor Information
(209) 372-0200

Appendix B:

Managing Agencies

SOUTH: AGNEW MEADOWS TO CA HIGHWAY 50

1. Agnew Meadows to Thousand Island Lake: Mammoth Lakes Visitor Center, Inyo National Forest
2. Tuolumne Meadows to Ireland Lake: Tuolumne Ranger Station, Yosemite National Park
3. Tuolumne Meadows to Waterwheel Falls: Tuolumne Ranger Station, Yosemite National Park
4. Sonora Pass to Leavitt Lake: Summit Ranger Station, Stanislaus National Forest
5. Sonora Pass to Sonora Peak: Summit Ranger Station, Stanislaus National Forest
6. Clark Fork to Disaster Creek: Summit Ranger Station, Stanislaus National Forest
7. Wolf Creek: Calaveras Ranger District, Stanislaus National Forest
8. Ebbetts Pass to Upper Kinney Lake: Amador Ranger Station, Eldorado National Forest
9. Carson Pass to Fourth of July Lake: Eldorado National Forest
10. Carson Pass to Winnemucca Lake: Eldorado National Forest
11. Carson Pass to Showers Lake: Eldorado National Forest

LAKE TAHOE AREA: CA HIGHWAY 50 TO INTERSTATE 80

12. Echo Summit to Meiss Meadows Overlook: Eldorado National Forest
13. Echo Lake to Lake Aloha: Lake Tahoe Basin Management Unit, Eldorado National Forest
14. Emerald Bay to Lake Aloha: Lake Tahoe Basin Management Unit, Eldorado National Forest
15. Barker Pass to Twin Peaks: Lake Tahoe Basin Management Unit

Index

INDEX

About the Author

AT AROUND THE TURN OF THE CENTURY, **Wendy Lautner** was a recovering pre-med major at Humboldt State University in beautiful Northern California. Having recently returned from a study-abroad program in Central America, she found the idea of sitting in one place for too long hard to fathom. When she discussed this dilemma with her father, he suggested she try journalism: "Then you can travel and do all kinds of fun things and get paid well for it."

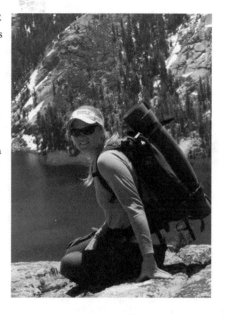

While she still hasn't mastered the getting-paid-well part, Wendy took her dad's wise advice and signed up for the school newspaper the next day. She has since worked at *Paddler Magazine* and written for a variety of newspapers and magazines in the Lake Tahoe and Sacramento areas covering a wide array of topics, including music and entertainment, sports, government, community issues, food, travel, and her favorite—recreation!